Eat Papayas Naked

The pH-Balanced Diet for Super Health & Glowing Beauty

By Susan M. Lark, M.D.

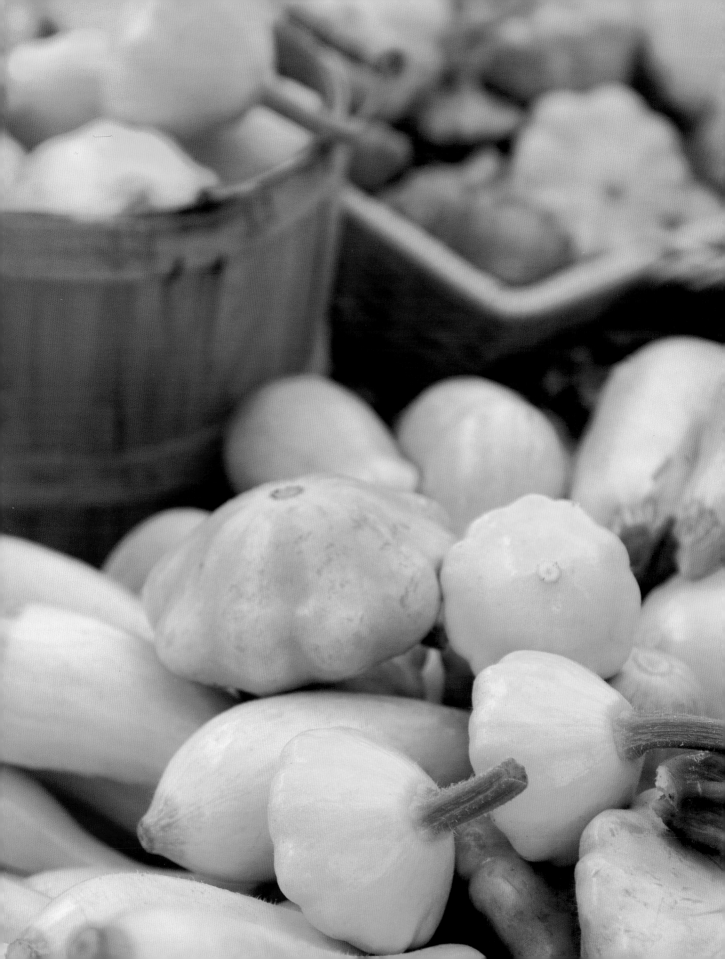

Table of Contents

5   Introduction

11 pHenomenal Balance for pHenomenal Health and Beauty
12 Determine Your Metabolic Type
13 pH Self Test
13 If You are Overly Acidic
16 If You are a High-Alkaline Producer
16 If You Easily Maintain an Acid and Alkaline Balance
17 Sneaky, Subtle Saboteurs
20 Take Back Your Vitality

23 Glowing Beauty
24 Rejuvenate Your Skin
24 Radiant, Youthful Skin
24 Treat Yourself Like a Queen
25 Avoid Dehydrating Foods
26 Erase Age Spots
26 Luscious Locks

29 Beauty Recipes
31 Shakes & Drinks
35 Snacks & Appetizers
43 Breakfast
53 Lunch
62 Dinner
71 Desserts

79 Natural Weight Loss

81   Rebalance Your Body

81   Eliminate False Fat

84   Rev Up Your Metabolism

85   Balance Blood Sugar

86   Rebalance Your Life

86   Exercise for Weight Loss

87   The Stress Connection

91 Weight Loss Recipes

92   Shakes & Drinks

99   Snacks & Appetizers

106   Breakfast

115   Lunch

124   Dinner

134   Desserts

140   The ABCs of Super Health and Glowing Beauty

145 Detox for Life

147   Take Out the Trash

147   The Original Multitasker

148   Toxic Backwash

148   My Love-Your-Liver Program

153 Detox Recipes

154   Shakes & Drinks

158   Snacks & Appetizers

165   Breakfast

172   Lunch

181   Dinner

190   Desserts

196 Appendix

196   pH of Common Foods

201 Index

Introduction

Think of this as a guidebook to a destination you've always wanted to visit—a place where you bask in your own skin, eating papayas, naked as the day you were born. I'm not advocating you get arrested for public nudity. I'm advocating that you make unprocessed, naked foods the cornerstone of your diet. Do this, and you'll not only be able to visit the land of *Eat Papayas Naked,* you'll be able to live here permanently—a place where foods are whole, ideally unprocessed, and full of nutrients. It's a place where being healthier, and looking and feeling younger and more radiant, are the daily fare. You can reach this destination by improving your body chemistry: By understanding how your body's pH affects your health, and how the food you eat affects your pH.

In this book, I'll help you identify on which side of the pH (acid/alkaline) spectrum your body falls, and the many ways this affects you. I'll show you how your food choices work for you—or against you—by tipping your body's pH toward better balance, or further off-kilter. I'll help you determine which foods you should eat more of, and which to de-emphasize. And, I'll give you practical, hands-on tips you can use every day: The best ways to prepare a particular food, for maximum impact, for example, and how to adapt your favorite old recipes with pH-balancing substitutions.

So you won't have to think about anything but the joy of eating good food that tastes heavenly, I'll also give you my collection of recipe favorites that are delicious, simple to prepare, beautiful to look at, and carefully crafted for pH balance and nutritional value that practically hums with vitality. Every dish on these pages is prepared with choice ingredients, such as fresh fruits and vegetables, wholesome grains, fresh herbs, and lean meats. You'll want to do your shopping at your favorite health food store, at your local farmers' market (my favorite choice of all), and around the perimeter of your grocery store (away from the dead, processed foods stacked like cordwood down the aisles). You'll see that there are no accidents in my recipes: Each ingredient is chosen not only for flavor and first-rate nutrition, but also for the chemistry of how it interacts within your body.

You'll feel different within just a few weeks, even if you didn't think there was anything "off" about the way you felt before. You'll also start to look younger and healthier. And, because you'll be eating the right foods, in the right amounts according to your body's particular makeup, you'll improve your overall health—not just looking and feeling better, but actually being better—by helping to decrease your risk for heart disease, coronary artery disease, high blood pressure, diabetes, chronic fatigue, PMS, and possibly even some kinds of cancer. And, by the way, you'll also notice that your clothes will get looser in all the right places, even though you'd given up on the prospect of ever losing those persistent extra inches.

Rome Wasn't Built in a Day

This isn't a "diet" in the boring, temporary, usually ineffective sense. It's a fresh new way of life, based on high-nutrient, low-stress, pH-balanced foods that'll entice you from the first bite, keeping you healthier, more energized, and brimming with a sense of well-being. It may seem like biting off more than you can chew, to permanently change a lifelong pattern of eating—especially if you've tried other diet plans, then fell back into your old ways. But look at it this way: It takes three weeks to form a new habit. So, take small bites of this new lifestyle—take it three weeks at a time. Within your first three weeks, you'll get so much encouragement from the way you look and feel that you won't look back, except to say, "I never knew what I'd been missing!" It comes down to this: Once you've set foot in the land of *Eat Papayas Naked,* you'll want to stay here for the rest of your life.

To help you make the transition, and make sure it sticks, I encourage you to take it slowly, and be skeptical. Don't take my word for anything; let the food prove itself to you. Ask friends and family to support you in this, and don't be surprised if they ask to join in (which usually comes after they've seen the changes in you). For now though, focus on you. Start gradually, introducing my recipes one at a time, and watch for the unmistakable bloom that will appear in your skin, the luster in your hair, the light in your eyes, and the boost in your physical energy and mental clarity. Even if you feel you already eat a healthy diet, I promise you that this book will give you new ways to let food carry you to a higher level of health and beauty.

A Healthy Trifecta

You may wonder why I've organized the heart of this book—the how-to section—into three separate programs: Glowing Beauty, Natural Weight Loss, and Detox for Life. That's because for the thousands of patients I've attended, these are by far the three biggest issues. Weight loss and beauty are at the top of every woman's list. And, from a physician's point of view, detox is a critical tool for redeeming and protecting our health against the daily barrage of toxic stresses, pollutants, food additives, metabolic by-products, and pharmaceuticals.

These three programs do have some crossover in their health advice and in the recipes I've designed for them. However, there are important differences as well. So, I've given each program a chapter of its own—with details about the foods that benefit that particular area, and recipes that use and enhance those foods—to bring it all to life for you. You don't need to follow (or even read) all the programs—just pick the one that best represents what you want to achieve first, and don't worry that you might be missing information from the other two. Rest assured, each program is built upon my pH-balance philosophy, with targeted guidance and recipes already balanced to the healthier, alkaline side. That way, no matter which program you choose, there'll be benefits across the board.

Choose beauty, for example, and in addition to gorgeous hair and a luminous complexion, you'll notice your waistband no longer pinches. Choose weight loss, and in addition to enjoying a slimmer body, you'll have younger looking, smoother skin. The detox program is the mother of them all: It amplifies everything positive. You'll enjoy a whole host of health benefits—obvious and behind-the-scenes—as you free your body of accumulated toxins. Your skin may break out during the first week or two on the program, when your body is kicking out old toxins through your pores, but in no time you'll see a glowing new complexion smiling back at you in the mirror. Plus, your hair will be thicker, glossier, more bountiful. It's like being reborn.

Why pH Matters

Your body has a built-in buffering system that's supposed to keep the pH level of your blood, cells, tissues, and intercellular fluids tipped slightly to the alkaline side. Your internal chemistry was designed to operate best in that mildly alkaline environment, for optimal digestion, keener immunity, stronger muscles, greater cardiovascular capacity, more efficient metabolism and enzyme reactions, more efficient cell growth and renewal, boundless energy...all the good stuff that goes with being radiantly healthy. This is what gave you a little-known chemical edge when you were young—able to eat terrible food, stay up all night, basically neglect yourself—and bounce right back.

That's because as acidifying as your diets and lifestyles may have been, your buffering system was able to handle your extreme behaviors, quickly adjusting and readjusting, bringing your body chemistry into balance—in spite of yourself. In modern adult life, we tend to continue the same sort of self-neglect in the form of highly acidifying foods, activities, stresses, and environmental factors. Unless you're one of the lucky ones born with a chemical edge, you may be marinating in your own acid right now.

The Chemical Edge

You can probably name a few people who are every bit as energetic and resilient and mentally sharp in their 60s, 70s, and 80s as they were in their teens. Tina Turner is one. Sophia Loren. Perhaps your Aunt Ellen, or your next-door neighbor's grandmother. The reason you notice these people is because they're extraordinary. They're among the select few of us who are what I call high alkaline producers: Able to maintain an alkaline pH—with the youthful vigor that goes with it—well into their senior years, even though they may still be living a stressful, high-energy lifestyle and eating all the "wrong" foods. In fact, they not only tolerate, but actually thrive, while burning the candle at both ends.

Despite strenuous overwork and less sleep, they get sick less often, recover faster, enjoy tremendous energy and stamina, and are more resilient overall. Their slightly alkaline makeup boosts their ability to have a positive, optimistic outlook, think on their feet, and get along with others, even in challenging social situations. When they pop out of bed in the morning, they hit the ground running—and smiling—and they consistently look and act younger than their age because, quite simply, they age more slowly. In old age, they tend to stay active and up-to-date on current world events, and they're more likely to live independently, right up to their final days—without a need for assisted living or a nursing home. They can do this because they're among the six to eight percent of us that were blessed with a more powerful and durable buffering system.

For the other 92–94 percent of us, our buffering system increasingly falters with age, and we begin to lose the chemical edge of our youth. What this means is that our body finds it more difficult to deal with the many influences in modern life that tend to acidify us. As we become more acidic, we become more vulnerable to such conditions as fibromyalgia, osteoporosis, chronic fatigue syndrome, chronic bladder infections, and rheumatoid arthritis. An acidic body pH is where aging sets its roots and changes everything: The way you feel, the way you function, and the way you look. The disadvantages of being overly acidic are daunting. They include fatigue; premature aches, pains, and wrinkles; increased body fat; reduced resistance to disease; and simply looking and feeling older than you are. The advantages of being a high-alkaline producer are nothing short of amazing!

Naked To The Rescue

If you weren't born with one of those rare, super-human buffering systems, but you'd love to feel younger, be healthier, and look more beautiful, then *Eat Papayas Naked* is for you. By choosing alkalinizing foods, and preparing them in a way that maximizes their pH-balancing power and nutritional punch, you can restore your pH balance to the slightly alkaline side for health and beauty benefits you may have thought were no longer possible. This book will make it all work for you by showing you how your diet drives your body's pH, and how your pH steers the quality of your life, so you'll be motivated to use the roadmap—those great recipes—that'll speed you to that fabulous destination we talked about. To help you choose your route, here's an overview of how the book is organized.

What You'll Find In Chapter 1: *pHenomenal Balance for pHenomenal Health and Beauty*

Chapter 1 is my secret weapon. It's how I motivate you to try my pH-balancing diet program. Yes, you'll love the flavors and the vitality of the dishes I'll help you prepare, but that doesn't mean you'll stick with the program. You're busy, and completely overhauling your relationship with food takes commitment. To motivate you, this chapter is meant to appeal to your intelligence, by helping you understand why and how my pH-balancing philosophy works. I'll make sure you understand what I mean by being acidic or alkaline, and I'll give you a little test to help you determine which one you are. Then, I'll show you how that seemingly tiny chemical characteristic affects the way you react to different kinds of food—and how that affects virtually everything in your life. I'll provide charts, showing where common foods fall on the acid/alkaline scale, and I'll give you some good substitutions for the foods you need to avoid. If your pH is seriously off balance, requiring an extra step to re-establish chemical harmony in your body, I'll walk you through a self-treatment method that will enhance the corrections made by the diet program you choose. In short, I'll give you the tools you need to remake your body chemistry into a system that rights itself, the way it did when you were young.

What You'll Find In Chapter 2: *Glowing Beauty*

If radiant skin and thick, shiny hair are your primary goal, restoring your pH balance through the guidance and recipes in Chapter 2 will do for you what no cosmetics, hair products, or even surgeon can do: Restore your body's ability to cleanse and invigorate your exterior from the inside, providing nutrient-rich blood to your skin and the follicles of your hair. The result: Moister, softer skin. Stronger, healthier hair. Simply beautiful in your natural, naked state.

What You'll Find In Chapter 3:
Natural Weight Loss

If you've been carrying extra weight around your middle, the guidance and recipes in Chapter 3 will help you get rid of the bloated, swollen tummy you've surrendered to. My program works, while typical weight-loss diets don't, because much of your stubbornly swollen midsection consists of false fat—a stagnant puddle of inflammatory fluids that are, in part, due to a diet that accelerates pH imbalance. Once your pH starts returning to a more balanced level, the false fat disappears. At that point, it becomes easier to eliminate excess real fat, as your blood sugar begins to come into balance, and your metabolism finds its second wind.

What You'll Find In Chapter 4:
Detox for Life

As your body's most overworked multi-tasker, your liver's most burdensome job is to dismantle and dispose of toxins in your body. Digesting and metabolizing even high-grade, wholesome food normally produces toxic by-products that your liver has to deal with—that's the reason we were born with a liver in the first place. Add modern-day toxins that were never part of the plan—air pollution, contaminated water, plastics, pharmaceuticals, mercury, lead, and so on—and your liver has to struggle to keep up with the workload. As a result, excess toxins build up in your system day in and day out. The toxins your liver can't manage to eliminate are stored in the body in various stages of breakdown—in the liver itself, in the skin, in the lungs, and in the body fat and intercellular spaces. Excess toxin storage in the body not only enables inflammation, false fat, "real" fat, and fluid retention, but it also can put you at elevated risk for cancer, heart disease, a weakened immune system, allergies, and so on. My detox program will help you give your liver a much-needed deep cleaning, and invigorate it by restoring pH balance through diet and lifestyle upgrades. Love your liver, and it will repay you many times over.

No matter what your age, no matter how you feel, whether you're happy with your looks or would like to see some improvement, there's no better time than right now for you to elevate your health and beauty to a whole new level. I hope you'll choose your Naked program today, and get started right away. You'll never be the same, and you'll be glad of it!

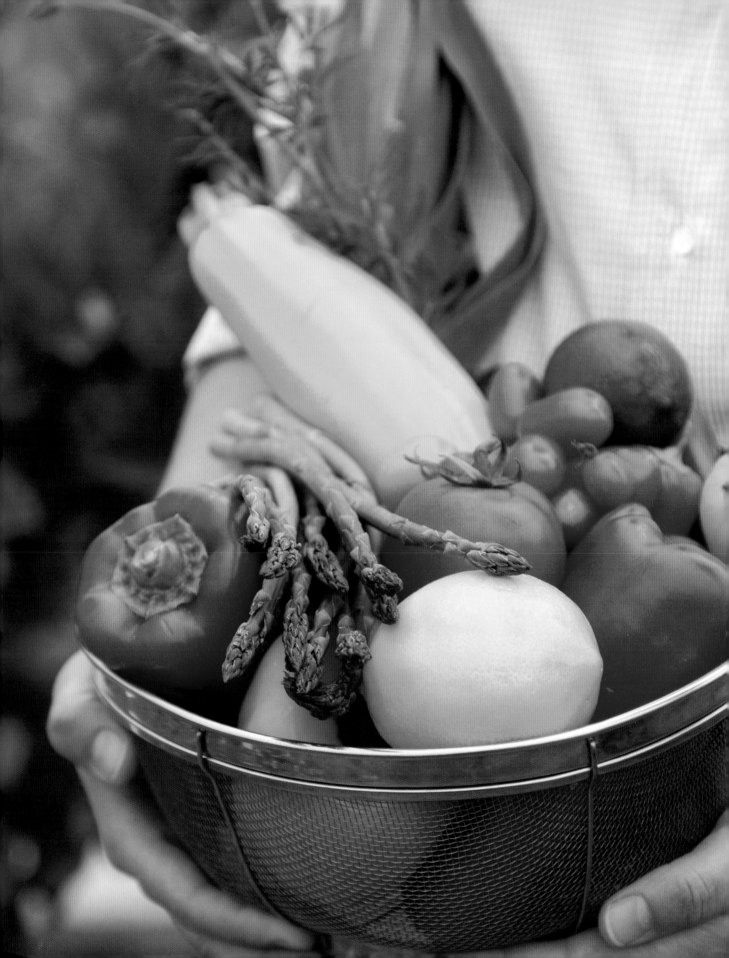

pHenomenal Balance for pHenomenal Health and Beauty

For many women, including myself, each day is a struggle to find balance in our lives. More and more of us work outside the home while continuing to meet the demands of family life. And, very often, we find ourselves in the role of primary caregiver, not only to our children, but also to our husbands, significant others, and even aging parents.

As we enter our 40s and 50s, we find that our energy levels are dropping and the juggling act is getting more difficult. For me, the key has been to lift my health to a higher level, so I can meet the demands of my busy life, and still engage in the activities that are just for me. In this book, I offer you the same solutions I use to restore my energy and regain the vitality necessary to really enjoy being alive. It's not just about keeping up with your workload; it's about feeling good, looking great, and enjoying a sparkling, vibrant kind of health you haven't experienced in so long, you've probably forgotten what it's like.

It's All About Balance

In its natural, healthy state, your body is slightly alkaline. What does that mean? It means your blood, tissues, cells, and intercellular fluids are slightly to the alkaline side of pure water. In pH terms, water is neutral, with a pH of 7. Anything that's acidic has a pH below 7—the lower the pH number, the stronger the acid. Anything with a pH higher than 7 is alkaline—the more alkaline it is, the higher the pH. Your very survival depends on your internal body chemistry's ability to keep you within a narrow pH range centered around that slightly alkaline goal. You have a built-in buffering system—your very own chemical juggler—to do just that. It measures, adjusts, and readjusts your pH to keep poor food choices, stress, pollutants, alcohol, and other external factors from upsetting your vital internal balance. I believe strongly that maintaining a healthy acid/alkaline balance, and eating pH-appropriate foods that are right for your body's chemical makeup, is the most powerful way to keep your health at peak levels.

However, for many of us, as we reach the age of 40 and beyond, our buffering system begins to falter, making it increasingly difficult to maintain that optimal pH. Virtually everything we're exposed to—from the foods we eat, the activities we engage in, and the pollutants we encounter—produces acidic chemicals. This tips us out of our ideal acid/alkaline balance and exposes us to a daunting list of physical and emotional ailments, including fatigue, headaches, chronic illnesses, colds, flu, and even an inability to think clearly. If, instead, you can maintain a healthy acid/alkaline balance, you can avoid many of those physical and emotional problems that plague the overly acidic person. And how do you achieve that balance? Largely through a diet like no other. Rather than counting calories, for this diet you simply need to eat top-quality, pH-balanced foods, in the right amounts (which will be easier, because these foods satisfy).

In this chapter, I'll lay the foundation for you, so you'll understand how the program works, and I'll tell you exactly what foods you need to eat. In the chapters that follow, you'll find more information about the foods that are best for you, and how to prepare them, with recipes that'll keep you luxuriating in delicious, simple-to-fix meals for a long time.

Determine Your Metabolic Type

Now that you know a bit about my philosophy on food and nutrition, it's time to focus on how you can bring your lifestyle into balance. Don't panic! Everything I'm going to suggest can be gradually and effortlessly integrated into your daily life at whatever pace feels right. The rewards will keep you moving forward. Let's start by figuring out where you are, so you can map out how to get where you need to be.

To determine if you are overly acidic or a high alkaline producer, you'll need to think about how your body reacts to different kinds of food. Take this self-test.

pH Self-Test: Are You Overly Acidic or a High-Alkaline Producer?

Check all phrases that apply to you in each section below. If you tend toward acidity, it's likely that you:

- ☐ Do not feel your best when you drink alcohol, coffee, or colas.
- ☐ Do not feel your best when you eat red meat or sugary desserts.
- ☐ Do not tolerate vinegar, citrus fruits, and white flour.
- ☐ Feel best when you eat a more vegetarian diet.
- ☐ Often feel exhausted after vigorous exercise or very physical work.
- ☐ Often experience fatigue and lack of stamina.
- ☐ Are physically and mentally tired after an hour of deskwork.
- ☐ Are subject to frequent flus, colds, bronchitis, or sinusitis.
- ☐ Are susceptible to heartburn, canker sores, and food or environmental allergies.

If you tend toward alkaline, it's likely that you:

- ☐ Have great physical endurance and can sprint up stairs easily.
- ☐ Are always on the go and full of energy.
- ☐ Need a few hours of sleep each night.
- ☐ Prefer highly active sports and gravitate toward high stress activities.
- ☐ Feel bright and energized after a steak dinner.
- ☐ Are able to digest a wide variety of foods.
- ☐ Feel de-energized after a low protein, high carbohydrate meal.
- ☐ Typically have lots of energy in the midst of intense situations.
- ☐ Are able to do deskwork for long hours at a time without becoming tired or losing mental clarity.
- ☐ Rarely get a cold or flu, and are free of allergies.
- ☐ Have a great digestive system.
- ☐ Are strong, with a large frame and big bones.

If You are Overly Acidic

I'm going to lay it right out on the table: If you're overly acidic, which describes more than 90 percent of the American population, the food you eat is a big part of the problem. The typical American diet is dominated by foods that are either highly acidic to begin with, or, once eaten, cause an acidic reaction within the body. This is likely to have contributed to your becoming acidic, and is definitely making it worse. And, because the acid/alkaline effects of foods are rarely, if ever, discussed by nutritionists and never included on labels,

even "health nuts" are likely to find—to their great surprise—that some of the "healthy" food choices they make are not in their best interest, pH-wise. Once you become overly acidic, you're at increased risk for developing environmental allergies, food intolerances, digestive upsets, respiratory ailments, low bone density, immune problems, and fatigue issues. The more acidic you become, the faster you'll age, the older and more tired you'll look, and the bigger your health risks.

What to do. If you are overly acidic, the first thing to do is avoid highly acidic and acid-forming foods as

Use the following chart to determine the kinds and quantities of foods you should be eating if you are overly acidic.

Grains	5-7 servings a day	Rice; Wild rice; Oats; Buckwheat; Corn; Millet; Quinoa; Amaranth Products made with any of these grains
Vegetables	4-6 servings a day	Bell peppers; Green leafy vegetables, such as lettuce and spinach; Carrots; Broccoli; Cauliflower; Potatoes; Onions; Celery; Mushrooms; Asparagus; Artichokes
Fruit	1-2 servings a day	Papaya; Mango; Figs; Avocados; Dates; Melon; Bananas; Pears
Legumes	At least one serving per day	Kidney beans; Pinto beans; Lentils; Soybeans; Peas; Garbanzo beans; Lima beans; Hummus; Tofu
Fish/Poultry	2-3 servings a week (4-ounce serving)	Salmon; Tuna; Trout; Mackerel; Free-range chicken or turkey ; Organic eggs; Shellfish; Oysters; Clams
Condiments	as needed	Molasses; Cocoa; Honey; Maple syrup; Bragg Liquid Aminos (similar to low-sodium soy sauce); Tamari sauce; Xylitol

much as possible, and try to get as many alkaline-enhancing foods into your diet as you can. Throughout this chapter, you'll find the pH values of many common foods. Remember, a pH of 7 is neutral, like water. Higher than 7 is alkaline—these are the foods you'll want to eat more of. Lower than 7 is acidic—the lower the pH, the stronger the acidity—these are the foods you'll want to avoid.

Overall, you should eat a predominantly vegetarian diet, choosing more alkaline sources of protein, such as fish, shellfish, tofu, eggs; legumes such as peas and beans; and breads made with non-wheat flours, like rice, millet, amaranth, quinoa, oat, corn, and buckwheat flours.

Use delicious and readily available substitutions for highly acidic foods, such as sugar-free ketchup in place of regular ketchup, green tea or herbal coffee replacements such as Teeccino instead of coffee, and baked corn and potato chips rather than fried. Plan more meals around vegetables and legumes, rather than meats, breads, and pastas made with white flour. And stay away from sugar, caffeine, and red or processed meats, which further acidify your body.

The Bicarbonate Boost

If you're overly acidic, an alkalinizing diet may not be enough at first—you may need to take an additional, more aggressive step, to restore your pH balance. For my patients, this applies to anybody who already has symptoms of being overly acidic, perhaps including a diagnosis such as osteoporosis, recurrent bladder infections, allergies, recurrent respiratory illnesses, fibromyalgia, depression, fatigue, etc. For these individuals, taking supplemental bicarbonate can bring accelerated symptom relief and help the alkalinizing diet restore balance faster.

What is Bicarbonate?

Bicarbonate is a natural alkalinizing substance that plays a critical role in your body's buffering system. Unfortunately, your natural supplies of bicarbonate can be pushed to their limit by a big, constant acidifying challenge. That's when your body's ability to maintain pH balance begins to fail, and the symptoms of an overly acidic constitution can appear. You're likely to look and feel older, begin losing your resistance to illnesses, suffer metabolic breakdowns such as osteoporosis, and find that you're prone to allergies that never bothered you before. Supplemental bicarbonate can work wonders by naturally restoring and supporting your buffering system's ability to do its job.

How To Take Bicarbonate

I generally recommend taking supplemental bicarbonate in a mixture of two parts sodium bicarbonate (baking soda), with one part potassium bicarbonate (must be purchased from a pharmacist). You can either ask a pharmacist to prepare the 2-to-1 bicarbonate mixture for you, or you can buy my pre-mixed product (Daily Balance Alkalinizer) by calling 888.314.5275 or ordering online at *www.drlark.com.*

Note: Potassium bicarbonate can be irritating to the gastrointestinal tract. If irritation occurs, stop taking it and use plain baking soda by itself.

A Word of Caution

Very occasionally, a person will take too much bicarbonate and become overly alkaline. While bicarbonate is perfectly safe for most people, you should observe the following precautions:

- If you're on a low-sodium diet under a physician's advice, and/or taking certain heart medications, and/or may be pregnant, you should not take large amounts of sodium bicarbonate. Ask your physician for guidelines.
- Potassium bicarbonate is not recommended for individuals who have a medical condition or take a medication that would make a potassium supplement inadvisable. Consult your physician.
- Too much bicarbonate can cause alkalosis—a state of excess alkalinity. The small amount of bicarbonate I recommend is highly unlikely to cause alkalosis. However, if you experience tingling in your arms, legs or lips, become anxious or panicky, or feel bloated or gassy, cut back on the amount of bicarbonate you take and how often you take it. For immediate relief of alkalosis symptoms, drink black coffee, black tea, or the juice of one-half lemon in water, and adjust your bicarbonate supplementation program.

Use the following chart to determine the kinds and quantities of foods you should be eating if you are a high-alkaline producer.

Grains	1–2 servings a day	Rice; Wild rice; Oats; Buckwheat; Corn; Millet; Quinoa; Amaranth Products made with any of these grains
Vegetables	4–6 servings a day	Tomatoes; Cucumbers; String beans; Peppers; Lettuce; Spinach; Carrots; Celery; Broccoli; Cauliflower; Potatoes; Onions; Asparagus
Fruit	2–4 servings a day	Oranges; Apples; Pineapple; All berries; Grapefruit ; Avocados; Melon; Bananas; Pears; Peaches; Cherries; Lemons; Limes
Legumes	1–2 servings a day	Kidney beans; Pinto beans; Lentils; Soybeans; Peas; Garbanzo beans; Lima beans; Hummus; Tofu
Fish/Poultry	2–4 servings a week (4-ounce serving)	Salmon; Tuna; Trout; Mackerel; Free-range chicken or turkey; Organic eggs; Shellfish; Oysters; Clams
Condiments	as needed	Vinegar; Pickles; Mayonnaise; Molasses; Cocoa; Honey; Maple syrup; Bragg Liquid Aminos (similar to low-sodium soy sauce); Tamari sauce; Xylitol

If You're a High-Alkaline Producer

A much smaller percent (about 6–8 percent) of the population are high-alkaline producers. They tend to be robust and hardy, and thrive on a busy lifestyle and intense exercise. Such people actually need a more acidic diet, in which meats can play a more prominent role. However, they need to steer clear of high levels of animal fat and sugar, which can lead to obesity, osteoarthritis, high blood pressure, heart disease, and reproductive cancers, such as breast and prostate cancer.

If you are a high-alkaline producer, your meals need to be higher in protein and lower in carbohydrates.

You can enjoy most fruits and juices, including citrus fruits and tomatoes, and use vinegar in your dressings. If your budget permits, you can meet some of your higher protein needs by including several servings of lean, range-fed beef, lamb, free-range poultry, or wild, cold-water fish each week.

If You Easily Maintain an Acid and Alkaline Balance

In our youth, most people are able to naturally maintain an optimal acid/alkaline balance, eating a wide variety of foods with few repercussions. However, once most women reach mid-life and older, they cannot continue to eat this way. If you are in the very rare category of women who can still easily maintain an acid/alkaline balance after menopause, then you are truly lucky.

To preserve this state of healthy balance, continue to eat a wide range of healthy, nutritious foods from both sides of the pH scale. You can even have red meat and other acidic foods as desired, but it'd be wise for you to give those foods a lesser role, and make my alkalinizing program the backbone of your diet. This will reduce your acid load and protect your buffering system from burnout. (I know buffer burnout can occur, because it happened to me many years ago!).

Just be sure to pay attention to any signs that you're tipping out of balance—such as fatigue, headaches, achey joints, or unusual weight gain (which could be related to false fat). If that happens, it's best to follow the recommendations for the overly acidic body type until your balance is restored.

Whichever category you fit—overly acidic, high-alkaline, or blessed with balance—your own personal version of the *Eat Papayas Naked* diet and recipes, found in Chapter Two, Three, or Four, will make it easy for you to restore and maintain optimal health. To choose the program for you, all you have to do is decide what you want the focus of your healthy upgrade to be: Enhanced beauty, weight loss, or detox. Then, go ahead—Get Naked!

Sneaky, Subtle Saboteurs

There are certain classes of food and drink you should limit or avoid, regardless of where you fall on the acid/alkaline scale. These foods have little, if any, nutritional value, and they may even cause you to lose valuable nutrients as your body processes them. The following is a list of the major offenders.

Alcohol

Numerous studies show that women metabolize alcohol more slowly than men do, thus alcohol's toxic effects remain longer in a woman's body. Also, because women are smaller and have a higher body fat content, the same size drink will concentrate more alcohol in a woman's body.

Because alcohol increases a woman's estrogen levels, it can inhibit ovulation and is associated with such health risks as endometriosis, heavy bleeding, and the development of breast cancer. For women in menopause, alcohol can worsen hot flashes and mood

> If you are taking conventional or natural hormones, or an anti-osteoporosis drug (such as Fosamax or Calcitonin), the alkalinizing diet won't interfere. In fact, just the opposite: A balanced pH can help you get better results, by supporting healthy bone in ways your medication can't. If you have been diagnosed with osteoporosis, or osteopenia (a silent decrease in bone mass that can only be detected by testing), and you're not already taking bicarbonate on a regular basis, I encourage you to make bicarbonate part of your daily routine, in combination with one of the alkalinizing diets in this book, for the sake of maximized mass and strength of your bones.

swings, and intensify menopausal fatigue and depression. It can impair heart muscle action and electrical conductivity, eventually leading to congestive heart failure, cardiac arrhythmias, and cardiac enlargement. Alcohol also can contribute its high sugar content to the feeding of the *Candida* fungus, resulting in even more mood swings and fatigue, as well as vaginal infections.

Tips:
If you want to enjoy a cocktail or glass of wine on occasion, don't drink on an empty stomach, which will absorb the alcohol almost immediately and overwhelm your liver's ability to metabolize and detoxify it. Instead, first eat some sort of oily or fatty food, such as a salad with an oil-based dressing or wild salmon. Better yet, skip the alcohol and have sparkling water with a lemon or lime twist.

Caffeine

If you habitually drink coffee or cola, or indulge in a chocolate bar every afternoon, the caffeine stimulates the release of excess stress hormones from your adrenal glands, increasing nervousness, anxiety and panic, and stealing valuable nutrients from the rest of your body to feed your overcharged, stressed nervous system. Caffeine can also increase estrogen levels, thus contributing to menstrual problems, breast pain, menopausal hot flashes, as well as certain cancers. It interferes with absorption of iron and calcium, while its diuretic effects cause other valuable vitamins and minerals to be lost in your urine. Plus, it raises blood levels of cholesterol and triglycerides, increasing your risk of heart disease; and increases acid production in the stomach, a risk factor for numerous types of gastrointestinal upsets.

Food Substitutes

Instead of...	Try...
Beef, veal, lamb, and pork	Wild fish and shellfish, free-range poultry, and occasional grass-fed red meat and game
Butter	Flaxseed oil, Spectrum Spread
Cheese	Rice and almond cheeses
Chocolate	Carob chips and bars
Coffee	Herbal coffee substitutes, such Teeccino, or herbal teas such as peppermint, chamomile, ginger, and rose hips
Cow's milk	Almond or rice milk, or milk made from oats or barley
Hamburger/hotdogs	Tofu or soy substitutes
Ice cream	Sorbet or frozen desserts made with rice milk
Margarine	Olive oil, fresh fruit preserves, raw seed and nut butters
Mayonnaise	Safflower or canola oil-based mayonnaise
Pizza made with wheat crust	Pizza made with rice flour crust and non-dairy cheese
Refined white sugar	Xylitol
Salt	Garlic, fresh herbs, sea vegetables, lemon rind, Bragg Liquid Aminos, miso
Soft drinks and fruit juices	Mineral water
Wheat products	Choose those made with rice, millet, amaranth, buckwheat, barley, corn, quinoa, oat, potato
Wheat cereals	Oatmeal, cream of buckwheat, quinoa or millet flakes, corn or rice flakes

Given all this, many women still balk at the idea of quitting caffeine "cold turkey," often unwilling to tolerate the unpleasant withdrawal symptoms, such as headaches, depression, and fatigue. That's why I've always recommended a gentle weaning process, by slowly decreasing the amount, and frequency, of your caffeine intake. Start by cutting both in half—reducing the size of your cup by 50 percent or "cutting" your coffee 50–50 with decaf, and replacing half of your "caffeine" breaks, whether they're in the form of coffee or chocolate or caffeinated soft drinks, with something healthy and naturally caffeine-free. Or, replace one break with a pleasantly brisk walk. Once you can comfortably maintain this level of caffeine reduction, reduce your intake by half again... and so on, until you've preserved the breaks, but replaced the caffeine.

Tips:
Experiment with an herbal coffee substitute, such as Teeccino. Try green or red tea instead of black varieties. For an afternoon pick-me-up, try a carob bar or piece of fruit instead of chocolate.

Dairy Products

Lactose intolerance—the inability to digest milk sugar—afflicts 30–50 million Americans and causes cramping, bloating, gas, diarrhea, and nausea. Even if you aren't allergic to—or intolerant of—dairy products, the artificial hormones and pesticides used in livestock feed make cow's milk an unhealthy choice. Whether you choose skim or full-fat, dairy products are one of the primary sources of food allergies in the Standard American Diet (SAD), causing such symptoms as fatigue, depression, bloating, intestinal

gas, bowel changes, wheezing, post-nasal drip, nasal congestion, and frequent colds. A lesser-known, delayed reaction to dairy manifests as anxiety, irritability, depression or mood swings, insomnia, fatigue, dizziness, confusion , disorientation, headaches, and joint pain. Dairy-related allergies can also make PMS symptoms worse, and weaken your adrenal glands over time, increasing your susceptibility to stress.

Tips:
Try almond or rice milk instead of dairy milk. Use "veggie slices" on your next sandwich instead of cheese. Buy sorbet rather than ice cream for a delicious frozen treat.

Sugar and Artificial Sweeteners

Sugar is a major source of dietary acid, with no vitamins or minerals left after processing—only simple glucose, which breaks down rapidly in your digestive system, producing acids. Sugar also makes your liver work harder to produce bile and other essential digestive enzymes.

Sugar contributes to blood sugar imbalances such as food cravings, insulin resistance, metabolic syndrome, and diabetes. It worsens PMS symptoms, anxiety irritability, and nervous tension. It also depletes levels of B-complex vitamins and valuable minerals. It intensifies fatigue by narrowing blood vessels, which makes your heart and lungs work harder to move blood through your body. And, it feeds the *Candida* fungus, leading to yeast infections and emotional symptoms like depression and nervous tension.

While you cannot control the amount of sugar that is automatically added to many foods, you can control your intake by eating Naked! Make natural, unprocessed foods the backbone of your diet, and refrain from adding sugar to foods such as cereal, oatmeal, homemade sweets, and tea, and you'll go a long way towards relieving your overburdened buffering system.

Tips:
Try healthier, unprocessed sweeteners such as raw honey or stevia instead of sugar in your tea. When baking desserts, try substituting all-natural xylitol (available at health food stores) for sugar. Sweeten your oatmeal with applesauce and raisins. Attack those sweet cravings with a bowl of fresh fruit topped with a spoonful of vanilla soy yogurt.

And, I have to warn you: As upsetting as sugar is to your acid/alkaline balance, artificial, chemical-based sweeteners create problems of their own. Most have no nutritional value and may worsen PMS and general anxiety symptoms. The key to breaking a sugar addiction isn't to replace it with artificial sweeteners. Rather, by making naturally sweet, naked foods the centerpiece of your diet, you'll gradually find that your sweet tooth is easier to satisfy than you thought.

Wheat and Gluten-Containing Grains

Like dairy, many women find they're intolerant of—or allergic to—wheat products. That's because wheat contains a protein called gluten, which is difficult for your body to break down, absorb, and assimilate. Women with wheat intolerance are prone to fatigue, depression, bloating, intestinal gas, bowel changes, post-nasal drip, nasal congestion, and frequent colds.

Are You Wheat or Gluten Intolerant?

Check all of the symptoms that apply to you.

__ fatigue   __ depression
__ bloating   __ intestinal gas
__ bowel changes   __ nasal and sinus
                       congestion

If you marked two or more items, you should eliminate all gluten-containing grains from your diet, including wheat, rye, and barley for at least one week to see if you feel a difference.

Even if you are not allergic, wheat can still trigger emotional symptoms and fatigue in women with PMS; intensify sinus and nasal congestion, particularly in women with allergies; and contribute to yeast infections, since wheat is leavened with yeast.

Tips:
Try pasta made from rice, corn, or buckwheat. Make corn bread rather than whole wheat bread to accompany your meals. Use bread made with rice, millet, or oat flour. Experiment with flaxseed crackers topped with tuna, sliced apple, almond butter, or hummus.

Take Back Your Vitality

Beauty and age are not mutually exclusive. This is a big revelation for a lot of women. Your outward appearance is a reflection of many things—your diet, environment, relationships, and lifestyle—and age takes a backseat to them all. If you take care of yourself, you'll regain the radiance and vitality you once had, and you'll keep that glow for life. By letting go of what our culture preaches about what happens when you age, you can write your own script to ensure that you stay healthy, happy, relaxed, and naturally beautiful. As you delve deeper into this book and, I hope, make gradual changes in your food choices based on your body's needs, you will grow ever closer to that healthy, happy, relaxed, and beautiful place, where you wouldn't dream of doing anything but *Eat Papayas Naked*.

Restaurant Rescue

It's difficult enough to control what you eat at home, but what about eating out? You may not be able to alter the amount of vinegar, citrus juices, etc., that the chef at your favorite restaurant uses. And, let's face it, sometimes you just want that bowl of chilled gazpacho or spicy chili.

Luckily, you can—in moderation—thanks to pH Choice granules from pH Sciences. A few shakes of this product over your food—citrus fruits, tomatoes, pickles, even juices—neutralizes up to 90 percent of the acid without changing the food's flavor! How much you need depends on what you're eating— for example, ¼ teaspoon over spaghetti sauce and orange juice, ⅛ teaspoon over vinaigrette dressing. You'll never even know it's on there!

I always keep a small bottle stashed in my purse for emergencies. If you would like more information about pH Choice granules or are interested in picking up a bottle for yourself, call 888.314.5275 or visit online at *www.drlark.com*.

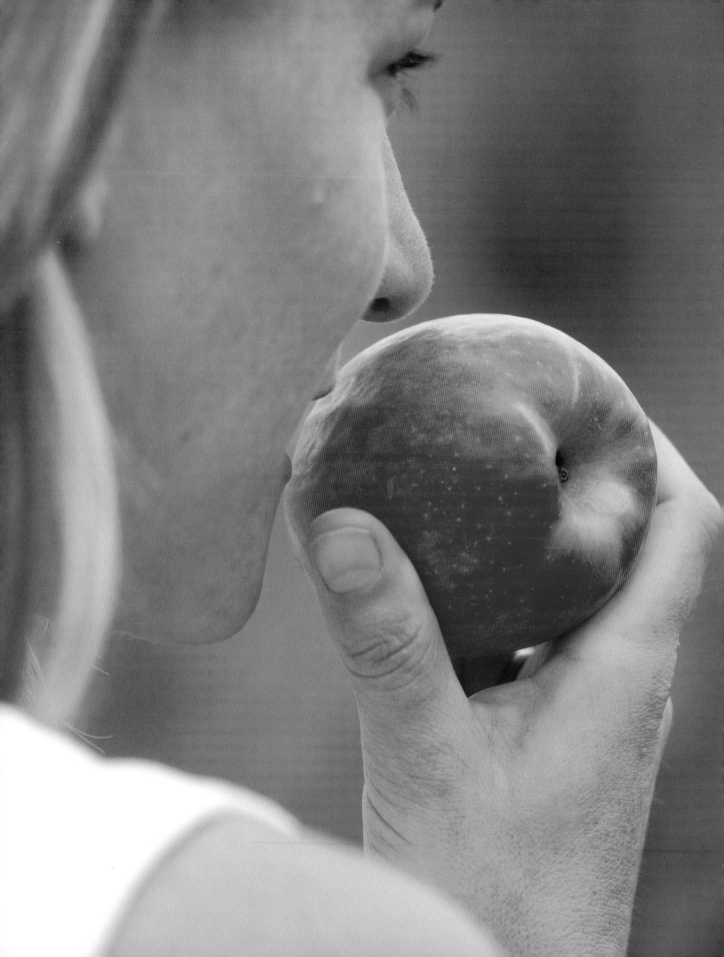

Glowing Beauty

Have you ever met a woman who, regardless of her age, just radiates beauty? If you look very closely, you'll be surprised to see that she may not have classically beautiful features, and she may not look as youthful as a teenager, but her skin is smooth, her hair gleams, her eyes shine, and she seems to light up every room she enters. We all know women like this and wonder…what's their secret?

I can tell you right now, it isn't makeup, moisturizers, peels, hair products, or the latest 'do. In fact, most of the so-called "beauty" products on the market are actually bad for your skin—and your health. The true secret is something every woman has been told since she was a little girl. Beauty is skin deep. In fact, it's deep in the cells of not only your skin, but your whole body. When you look good, you feel good. And when you feel good, you look good. That's because radiant beauty is the product of radiant health, and no amount of cosmetic diddling can fool the eye of the beholder for very long.

Rejuvenate Your Skin

Nothing betrays a woman's age like the drying and wrinkling of the sensitive and exposed skin on her hands, face, and neck. We blame it on age, but it's more than that. The damage to our skin gets accelerated and accentuated by improper nutrition, stress, lack of exercise, and hormonal changes that occur in midlife and beyond. No amount of moisturizer and sunscreen on the outside can remedy the deficits that develop in our skin's internal structure and health. To fill those holes, you need to focus on what's missing, and why.

Radiant, Youthful Skin

Proper hormonal support is essential throughout life for a woman to have healthy, moist, and resilient skin. Estrogen is responsible for the light cushion of fat under your skin, which gives you the soft, fine-textured glow we all enjoy in our younger years. Estrogen also preserves a healthy level of fluid and salt in the skin, which helps keep it plumped up and filled out.

During your reproductive years, your body produces enough estrogen to properly support the structure of your skin, but you lose much of this support as you go through menopause, when estrogen levels drop significantly. After menopause, your skin tends to gradually become thin and dry, and the underlying muscle and fat tissues that help to give skin its support begin to shrink. As a result, wrinkles and creases begin to become apparent and pronounced.

Unwilling to take hormones? Good. I don't prescribe them, except for a select few cases. But, there are many safe, natural, alternative therapies available that have a pronounced estrogen-like effect on your tissues, at much lower potencies and without the side effects of harsh synthetic hormones. Key among these great alternatives is soy. I recommend eating soy foods (such as tofu, tempeh, and soybeans). The gentle, plant-based estrogen in soy can give your aging skin a youthful estrogen boost, for a younger, plumper, filled-in appearance.

Treat Yourself Like a Queen

Using the Asian model, women are thought to become "yin deficient" when they reach menopause and their tissues become drier and hotter. Yin refers to the fluids and tissues of the body, as well as its structure, including the flesh, tendons, and bones. Traditional Asian medicine uses healing substances to restore or rebuild the yin, such as royal jelly—the food of the queen bee. I recommend taking ¼ teaspoon of liquid royal jelly twice a day. Royal jelly can be purchased at most health food stores. Women who are allergic to bees or have asthma should not take royal jelly or other bee products such as pollen.

A House Plant with Punch

Aloe vera—a simple, succulent house plant—also nurtures the yin with its ability to soothe, heal, and moisturize skin through external use, as well as taking it internally. There is a large body of research that documents the external use of aloe for a variety of dermatologic conditions, including rashes, acne scars, dermatitis, psoriasis, burns, and wound healing. It reduces the scaliness, itchiness, and extent of seborrheic dermatitis; prompts the remission of psoriasis; relieves poison ivy; assists the healing of chronic leg ulcers; and speeds healing after dermabrasion.

I recommend drinking 2–4 ounces of aloe vera juice per day, either mixed with water or juice, or blended in a smoothie. The juice is available at health food stores. In some cases, aloe vera can cause diarrhea. If this happens to you, reduce your intake until you can tolerate it comfortably.

Avoid Dehydrating Foods

The dehydrating effects of smoking, as well as many foods, dry out your skin and thin the underlying tissues—accelerating the very aging effect we want to slow, stop, and even reverse. Examples of dehydrating foods include spicy foods like ginger and chili peppers, caffeinated beverages, salty foods, and alcohol. If you are in midlife and beyond and have already noticed increased drying of your skin due to menopause-related hormone deficiency, you should be especially cautious in eating these foods. Refined sugar also accelerates skin aging by constricting capillaries in the skin, decreasing circulation there.

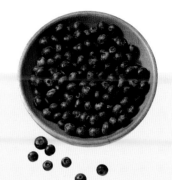

Antioxidants and Skin

Foods such as blueberries, cantaloupe, spinach, romaine lettuce, and broccoli are high in vitamins A, C, and E—powerful antioxidants that help to improve the overall health of your skin, specifically working to prevent ultraviolet light-induced inflammation, dryness, and damage to the skin.

Each vitamin benefits your skin in different ways. Vitamin A is especially helpful in suppressing oily skin and acne. In fact, one study found that high doses of vitamin A helped to clear up even the most severe cases of acne in 90 percent of the people treated with the vitamin.

Vitamin C works at a different level. It is needed for collagen production, thereby helping to strengthen the connective tissues underlying the superficial layer of the skin. It also has antiviral and antibacterial properties, which enhance your immune function by supporting white blood cell activity and increasing antibody levels. Plus, it has an antihistamine effect, which can help women whose allergies get worse just before their periods.

Finally, vitamin E is useful for a wide variety of dermatological complaints, including hyperpigmentation, warts, herpes, keloids, and atopic dermatitis. Through its ability to strengthen your immune system and its response to attack, vitamin E works to prevent cell damage throughout your entire body. It also has powerful antihistamine properties that can help you if you suffer from allergies.

Women with certain medical problems, such as high blood pressure and insulin-dependent diabetes, should begin taking vitamin E at lower doses, starting with 100 IU per day and slowly increasing the dose to the recommended levels.

Erase Age Spots

Sometimes called liver spots, age spots are the harmless, round or oval, flat, irregularly-edged brownish spots on the skin that begin to show after menopause. They're caused by an accumulation of debris in skin cells, due to free radical oxidative damage occurring throughout your body. Exposure to the sun's ultraviolet rays, heat, trauma, radiation, heavy metals, and changes in oxygen potential also affect the formation of melanin—the dark pigment in skin—and hasten the formation of age spots. And, according to Chinese medicine, dairy foods, red meats, and saturated fats congest your liver, blocking the chi (energy) and preventing your liver from detoxifying the blood. The result: Age spots, acne, eczema, boils, and other types of skin lesions.

Age spots usually accompany other symptoms of skin aging such as sagging, rough texture, and wrinkling. You may also have hypopigmentation—white spots—or other types of hyperpigmentation, such as freckles. These are all signs that the melanin-making mechanism is aging. I have found that the best way to treat age spots is from the inside, with the following natural remedies:

→ Research has shown that high vitamin A intake can significantly reduce the appearance of age spots. I suggest consuming 2–4 heaping teaspoons of spirulina (a greens food) a day. (One heaping teaspoon provides 10,000 IU of vitamin A.) You can also combat free radical damage with foods rich in beta-carotene, such as kale, spinach, squash, sweet potatoes, mangoes, cantaloupe, apricots, carrots, and cabbage.

→ Increase your intake of collagen-building vitamin C by eating foods such as cantaloupe, oranges, mangoes, blackberries, broccoli, and cauliflower.

→ Still smoking? Stop! It hastens the aging of your skin and contributes to free radical damage throughout your body.

→ Use sunscreen, at least SPF 15, whenever you go outside. It's never too late to start protecting your skin from the harmful effects of ultraviolet light.

Luscious Locks

In order for hair to grow thick and healthy, it needs a constant, nutrient-rich supply of blood to its follicles. I have found that a healthy hair diet includes adequate amounts of essential fatty acids (EFAs), zinc, copper, B vitamins, and selenium.

To ensure that you are getting enough EFAs in your diet, eat foods rich in omega-3 and omega-6 fatty acids, like flaxseed oil (1–2 tablespoons per day), flaxseeds (4–6 tablespoons per serving), and cold-water fish, such as salmon, trout, or halibut (3 times a week).

You also need to be sure that you are getting enough zinc in your diet. The best food sources for zinc are wheat germ, oysters, pumpkin seeds, and high-protein foods, such as chicken breast, eggs (especially organic, omega-3—rich eggs), and fish.

And don't forget the often overlooked mineral, copper, which helps form collagen in your hair. The best food sources for copper include seafood (especially

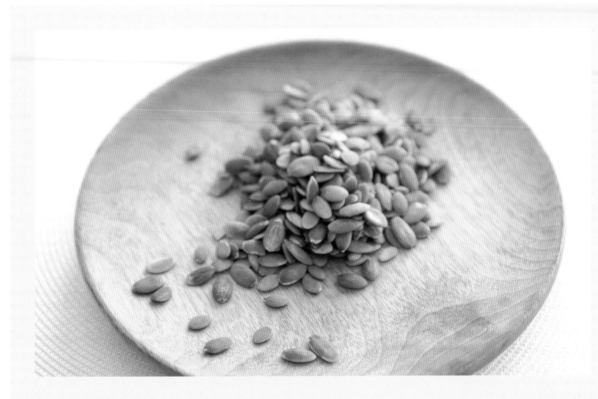

EFAs = Extremely Flawless Appearances

Olive oil is a great source of essential fatty acids (EFAs), fats that your body does not produce and that you must therefore obtain through diet or supplementation. EFAs help to substantially lower your risk of heart disease by lowering LDL cholesterol and triglycerides, preventing blood platelets from becoming sticky, and lowering blood pressure. They also help with bone health, heart health, and depression. A number of my patients have also had great results using essential fatty acids (EFAs) to create moister, softer skin and shinier hair.

Another reason I am particularly partial to olive oil is its squalene content. Squalene is a powerful natural antioxidant found in all human tissues, with the greatest concentration in the skin. It also has wonderful moisturizing benefits.

The moisturizing effect of these oils has been particularly evident in my younger patients who already have a high moisture content in their skin, so the beneficial effects are noticed much more quickly than with older women. For women at midlife and older who tend to have drier skin to begin with, it takes a little longer to replenish the moisture content. The process may take as long as three to six months.

To ensure that you are getting enough EFAs in your diet, eat foods rich in omega-3 and omega-6 fatty acids, like flaxseed oil (1–2 tablespoons per day), raw pumpkin seeds (2–3 ounces per serving), and cold-water fish, such as salmon, trout, or halibut (3 times a week). Be sure to include monounsaturated oils, like olive oil, in your diet. Use these oils in your salad dressing recipes and when cooking overall to help you moisturize your skin.

raw oysters), nuts, legumes, bran cereals, fruits and vegetables, and blackstrap molasses.

For rich sources of B complex vitamins, you can turn to a variety of foods, including chickpeas, bananas, and romaine lettuce. Other good food sources of vitamin B complex are brewer's yeast, beans, peas, kelp, mushrooms, whole grains, nuts, and seeds.

Finally, to increase your intake of selenium, be sure to include egg yolks, seafood, whole grains, lean red meats, chicken, and mushrooms in your diet.

Keep all of these focused tips in mind as you use the following recipes to create your meals. Based on a foundation of health-restoring pH balance through carefully chosen, top quality foods rich in all the right nutrients, each dish has been tailor-made to lift your health to a vibrant new level with an accent on youthful beauty.

Beauty Recipes

The following recipes contain many of the ingredients that will boost the beauty quotient of your skin, hair, and nails—as well as your overall well-being—with delicious results.

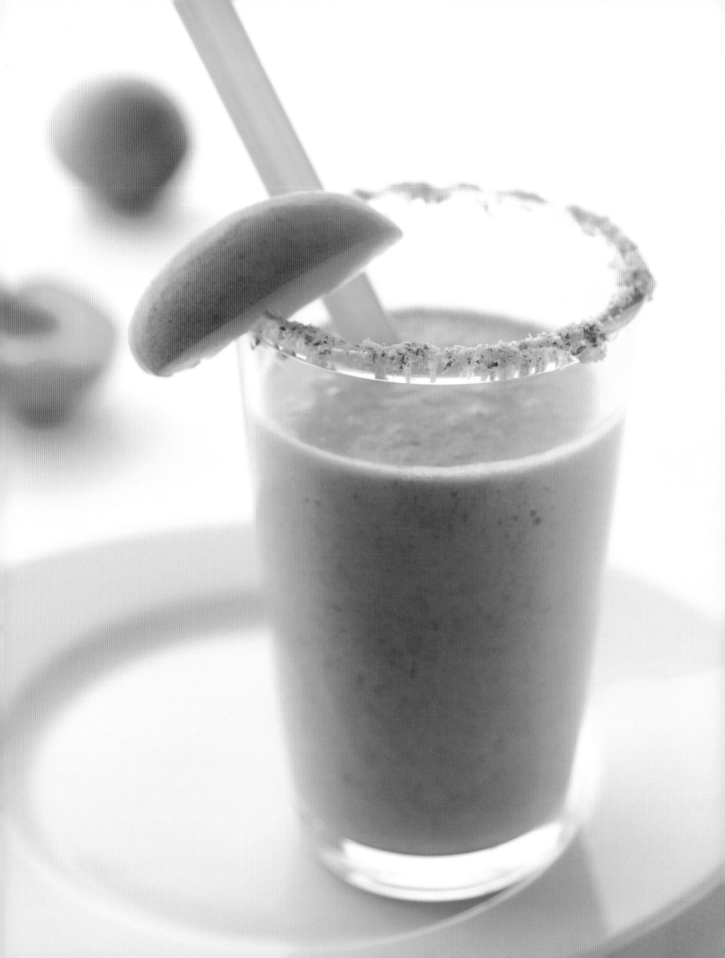

Shakes & Drinks

Apple-Nut Smoothie Serves 2

Apricots feature pantothenic acid, the beauty vitamin, plus silicic acid, which strengthens connective tissue, thus firming skin.

    4–6 fresh apricots (about 5 ounces)
    2 tablespoons apple juice concentrate
    4 teaspoons almond butter
    1 ⅓ cups cold almond milk
    3 tablespoons rice protein powder
    2 teaspoons vanilla extract
    ⅛–¼ cup ground almonds

Wash, halve, and pit the apricots, setting aside two apricot wedges as garnish. Put the remaining fruit, coarsely chopped, in blender with apple juice concentrate, almond butter, and half the almond milk. Blend well for 15–20 seconds. Add the remaining milk, rice protein powder, and vanilla, and flash-blend to smooth liquid.

Place ground almonds on a saucer or small, shallow dish. Moisten the rims of two large glasses with water, upturn the glasses, and dip the rims into the ground almonds. Put ice cubes in the glasses and pour in the smoothie blend. Cut slices into the reserved apricot wedges and decorate the glass rims with them. Serve the drinks with fat straws.

Avocado Fruit Shake Serves 2

Avocados provide unsaturated fatty acids for great skin, mannoheptulose for lowering blood pressure, and vitamin E to protect the heart.

- 1 small, soft avocado
- 2 sprigs fresh mint
- 1 ½ teaspoons fresh lemon juice
- 3 ½ tablespoons white grape juice
- 1 ¼ cups pear juice
- 1 teaspoon borage oil

Cut the avocado in half, remove the pit, and scrape the flesh out with a spoon. Clean and shake dry the mint, and remove the leaves from the stalks.

In a blender, purée the avocado, mint leaves, lemon juice, grape and pear juices, and borage oil. Add ice-cold water to taste.

Black Currant-Banana Blend Serves 2

Bananas contain high amounts of serotonin, which helps with resistance to stress and is a great mood enhancer.

- 1 medium banana
- 1 tablespoon lemon juice
- 4 teaspoons clover or sage honey
- 1 ½ cups black currant juice
- 2 tablespoons ground flax

Peel the banana, chop coarsely, and place in a blender. Add lemon juice, honey, and half of the currant juice. Blend well for 15 seconds. Add the ground flax and the remaining juice and blend for another 10 seconds.

Place ice cubes in a tall glass and pour the blend over the top.

Mango-Aloe Soother Serves 2

This drink is loaded with beta carotene and vitamin C.

    6 tablespoons aloe vera juice
    3 pieces mango (about 12 ounces)
    1 teaspoon borage oil
    1 tablespoon oat bran

In a blender, combine the aloe vera juice, mango, oil, and oat bran. Blend well at the highest speed.

Pour into tall glasses and serve immediately.

Mango-Carrot Cocktail Serves 2

Mangoes are rich in folic acid, which is necessary for the production of healthy red blood cells; while vegetarian protein powders, such as the rice protein powder called for below, usually contain both legume- and grain-based protein sources.

    2 pieces mango (about 8 ounces)
    1 tablespoon lime juice
    4 teaspoons clover or sage honey
    1 ½ cups cold carrot juice
    ¼ cup rice protein powder
    ¼ teaspoon ground ginger
    4 carrot strips (use a vegetable peeler)

Peel the mango, and cut a wedge for garnish and set aside.

Chop the remaining mango and place in a blender. Add the lime juice, honey and half the carrot juice, and blend for 15 seconds. Add the remaining carrot juice, protein powder, and ginger and blend well for another 10 seconds.

Place ice cubes in a large glass and pour the mixture into the glass. Place the mango wedge and carrot strips on the rims of the glasses, and serve cold.

Mocha Shake Serves 2

Daily consumption of honey raises blood levels of protective antioxidant compounds, while bee pollen contains concentrated nutrients, enzymes, and bioactive substances.

  2 ½ cups almond milk
  1 tablespoon Teeccino or other herbal coffee
  1 teaspoon Dagoba or other high-quality, organic cocoa powder
  1 teaspoon bee pollen
  1 tablespoon oats
  2–3 tablespoons honey
  1 finger banana (optional)

Add the milk, instant decaf coffee, cocoa powder, pollen, oats, and honey in a blender. Blend together until the ingredients are smooth and dissolved.

For a milder flavor and as an additional nutrient, try adding the banana.

Persimmon-Mango Cooler Serves 2

Rich in beta carotene and vitamin C, persimmons are an exotic and great-tasting fruit anytime.

  1 fully ripe Hachiya persimmon (about 8 ounces)
  1 ½ teaspoons lime juice
  ⅓ cup apple juice concentrate
  2 teaspoons vanilla extract
  3 pieces mango (about 12 ounces)
  2 tablespoons ground flax
  1 sprig fresh mint

Wash the persimmon and peel, remove core, and chop.

Place the persimmon, lime juice, and apple juice concentrate in a blender. Add the vanilla extract and half of the mango. Blend the mixture well for 15 seconds. Add the ground flax and the remaining mango and blend for another 10 seconds.

Pour the mixture into a large glass. Garnish with fresh mint.

Snacks & Appetizers

Apricot Corn Flake Muffins Makes 12

Apricots are rich in vitamin A, which quenches free-radical damage to tissue and cells and is especially helpful in suppressing oily skin and acne.

8 dried apricots
2 medium carrots
2 eggs
¼ cup honey
2 tablespoons raisins
1 ½ cups chopped almonds
Grated zest from ½ orange
⅔ cup rice flour
3 ½ tablespoons potato starch
5 ¼ teaspoons tapioca starch
2 teaspoons baking powder
Oil for the muffin pans
2 tablespoons apricot jam
2 tablespoons water
⅓ cup corn flakes

Preheat oven to 400°F. Thinly slice apricots into strips. Grate the peeled carrots and mix with the eggs and honey. Stir in raisins, apricot strips, almonds, and orange zest.

Sift together flour, potato and tapioca starches, and baking powder, then sift the flour into the apricot mixture, and stir until a stiff batter forms.

Lightly oil the muffin pans and spoon in the batter to no more than two-thirds capacity, as the batter will rise during baking. Smooth the tops. Bake in the middle of the preheated oven for about 20 minutes, until tops are golden brown.

While the muffins are baking, mix together in a small pot the apricot jam and water and warm slowly over medium-low heat until fluid. When muffins are done baking, cool them slightly on a rack, then brush muffins with apricot jam glaze, and sprinkle corn flakes on top, pressing lightly to adhere.

Banana-Hazelnut Muffins Makes 12

Vitamin E- and EFA-rich nuts also raise your spirits with their tryptophan, from which you produce the youth hormone melatonin and the mood-balancing hormone serotonin.

¼ cup plus 1 tablespoon honey
4 ounces Spectrum Spread
2 eggs
2 bananas
About 2 ounces ground hazelnuts
1 teaspoon vanilla extract
1 cup rice flour
⅓ cup potato starch
2 tablespoons plus 2 teaspoons tapioca starch
2 teaspoons baking powder
Oil for the muffin pans
About ¼ cup raisins
2 tablespoons maple syrup

Preheat the oven to 400°F.

In a medium bowl, with double-bladed mixer, blend ¼ cup honey, Spectrum Spread, and eggs for 5 minutes until light and foamy. Peel and mash the bananas. Add the mashed bananas, hazelnuts, remaining 1 tablespoon honey, and vanilla and blend for another 2 minutes until lightly creamy.

Sift the flour, potato and tapioca starches, baking powder, then sift the flour into the banana mixture, and stir in thoroughly.

Lightly oil the muffin pans and spoon in the batter to no more than two-thirds capacity, as the batter will rise during baking. Sprinkle the muffin tops with raisins, and bake them on the center rack of the preheated oven until golden brown, about 20 minutes.

Let cool completely in the pans and then brush muffins evenly with maple syrup.

Bean Dip with Leeks Serves 3–4

Beans contain fiber as well as fair portions of skin-protecting vitamin A and skin-firming vitamin C, while leeks, a member of the alum family with all onions and garlic, are known for their cleansing and detoxifying properties.

1 small leek
1 medium carrot
1 tablespoon olive oil
½ cup vegetable stock
1 small can pinto beans (8.75 ounces), drained
2 tablespoons minced fresh thyme (or 2 teaspoons dried, crumbled thyme)
2 teaspoons capers, drained
Salt to taste
Black pepper to taste

Trim the leek and carrot. Split leek lengthwise, wash, then slice crosswise into half rings. Peel and cut carrot into coin-shaped slices.

In a nonstick skillet, heat the olive oil and lightly sauté the vegetables over low heat for 10–15 minutes, until the stock has evaporated and the vegetables are tender-crisp.

Purée the pinto beans with the thyme, capers, leek, and carrot. Season the mixture with salt and pepper, then refrigerate.

This is a tasty dip for raw vegetables, but also works well as a spread for whole-grain or seed bread. Refrigerated, it keeps well for as long as a week.

Steamed Artichokes with Avocado Dip Serves 2

Artichokes contain cyranine, a powerful substance that stimulates the liver, thereby cleansing the blood. It also promotes cell renewal, giving your skin a radiant glow.

2 large artichokes
2 cups water
Dash of honey
Dash of cider vinegar
1 bunch fresh basil
1 ripe avocado
1 tablespoon fresh lemon juice
1 teaspoon olive oil
Sea salt to taste
White pepper to taste

After rinsing, scissor off the artichokes' tough, thorny tips. Snap or slice off the stem.

Bring the water to boil with the honey and vinegar. Cook the artichokes in the boiling water for about 30 minutes, until you can easily pull out a leaf. Remove the artichokes and reserve the cooking liquid. Wash and pat dry the basil (or use a salad shaker), and remove the leaves from the stems. Halve the avocado and remove the pit.

In blender or food processor, purée the avocado flesh with a little of the artichoke cooking liquid, the basil leaves, and the lemon juice. Stir in the olive oil. Season the dip with salt and pepper, and serve as an accompaniment to the warmed or cooled artichokes.

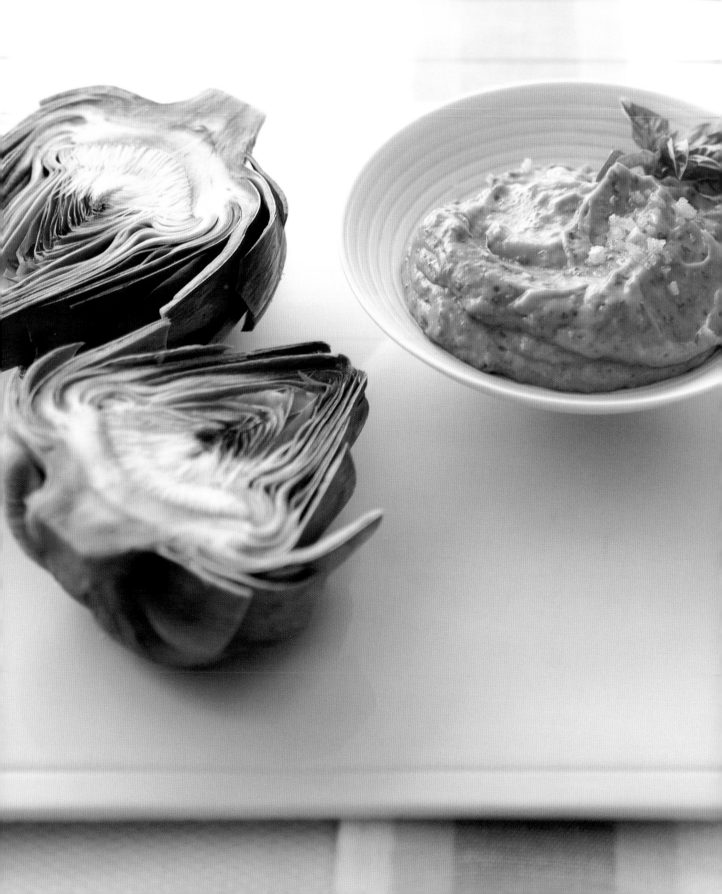

Pepita Salsa Verde Serves 2

This salsa contains alkaline-forming olives, as well as pumpkin seeds, an excellent source of iron and omega-3 and omega-6 fatty acids.

1 bunch fresh Italian parsley
1 bunch fresh cilantro
2 ounces pumpkin seeds (also known as pepitas)
2 ounces green olives, pitted
½ cup vegetable stock
2 tablespoons olive oil
Salt to taste
Black pepper to taste
1 clove garlic

Wash the herbs, pat dry (or use a salad shaker), and pull off the leaves.

In a food processor, purée the basil and parsley leaves with the pumpkin seeds and olives, and gradually add the stock. Mix in the oil and season with salt and pepper. Peel and finely chop the garlic and stir into the salsa.

Dairy products cause allergic reactions in many women, such as nasal congestion, swollen glands, and sore throat. As with wheat, dairy products can also lead to inflammation, which can also manifest as puffiness, especially in your eye area.

Tips:
→ Substitute cow's milk with soy milk, rice milk, or nut milk.
→ Use soy or rice cheeses—look for casein-free brands—instead of traditional cheeses.
→ Instead of milk-fat butter, substitute with flaxseed oil or almond butter for a spread, and olive oil for cooking.
→ Use "Veggie Slices" on your next sandwich instead of cheese.
→ Buy sorbet rather than ice cream for a delicious frozen treat.

Tuna Cream on Oatmeal Toast Serves 2

Tuna is one of the best sources of EFAs, while oatmeal is a super source of heart-friendly fiber.

    1 can water-packed tuna (6 ounces)
    1 tablespoon lemon juice
    2 tablespoons dairy-free sour cream or yogurt
    Salt to taste
    Black pepper to taste
    4 slices oatmeal bread
    4 radishes
    2 tablespoons minced fresh chives

Thoroughly drain the tuna in a sieve, and use a hand blender to purée the tuna with the lemon juice and sour cream or yogurt. Season with salt and pepper.

Toast the bread and spread with the tuna mixture. Wash and slice the radishes and arrange on top of the bread.

Sprinkle with chives and serve.

Turkey Prosciutto-Mushroom Appetizer Serves 2

Mushrooms are a good source of potassium, riboflavin, and selenium, which may help slow the growth of breast cancer cells.

About 2 ounces mushrooms
1 teaspoon fresh lemon juice
About 2 ounces turkey prosciutto or turkey ham, thinly sliced
¼ cup dairy-free cream cheese (e.g., Soya Kaas or Tofutti)
2 tablespoons minced fresh chives
2 thick slices wheat-free brown bread
Freshly ground black pepper to taste

Wash the mushrooms, dice them finely, and sprinkle with the lemon juice.

Remove excess fat from the prosciutto, cut the meat into confetti-sized pieces, and mix it with the mushrooms. Fold in the cream cheese and minced chives.

Spread the mixture onto the bread slices, garnish with fresh-ground pepper, and serve.

Breakfast

Almond Muesli with Diced Mango and Figs Serves 2

This breakfast dish is a rich source of magnesium and potassium, while figs are a fruit source of calcium, which promotes bone density.

About 2 ounces dried figs
3 tablespoons whole-grain oatmeal
¼ cup almond milk
¼ cup slivered almonds
⅔ cup diced mango, peeled
⅔ cup dairy-free yogurt
Pinch of ground cinnamon

Finely chop the figs, then mix with oatmeal and milk in a bowl, and let stand for 5 minutes.

Toast the almonds in a dry nonstick skillet.

Fold the mango and yogurt into the muesli mixture. Sprinkle with the toasted nuts and cinnamon before serving.

Apple-of-Your-Eye Pancakes Serves 2–3 (makes 4 or 5 pancakes)

Oats feature selenium, which contributes to healthy skin and nails, and silicic acid, which firms tissues and strengthens skin and hair, while the apples contain quercetin, a powerful antioxidant.

1 medium apple, peeling optional
2 egg whites
2 tablespoons oat flour
½ teaspoon cinnamon
½ teaspoon vanilla
2 slices oat bread
½ cup rice or nut milk
½ teaspoon baking soda
Olive oil spray, as needed
Applesauce or maple syrup to taste

Wash and halve the apple, cutting one half into chunks, the other into thin slices for garnish. Put the apple chunks into a blender or food processor with egg whites, oat flour, cinnamon, and vanilla. Blend until apple is well puréed. While food processor is puréeing, add torn bits of bread and milk alternately. Finally, add soda and continue to blend for a full minute until smooth.

On a hot pancake griddle coated with olive oil spray, spoon or ladle enough batter to spread into a 6-inch circle about ¼-inch thick. Allow pancake to brown on one side, then flip to brown other side. On same griddle, lightly sauté apple slices to garnish pancakes.

Top with applesauce or maple syrup.

Buckwheat-Apple Granola   Serves 2

This "stick-to-your-ribs" breakfast is loaded with gamma-linoleic acid, which contributes to healthy, firm skin.

2 ounces buckwheat groats
2 apples
2 tablespoons oat bran
5 tablespoons oat flakes
2 cups dairy-free yogurt
1 teaspoon borage oil
3–4 tablespoons maple syrup

Toast buckwheat in a dry, nonstick skillet over medium heat, until you begin to smell it.

Grate the washed and dried apples coarsely (do not peel). Mix the grated fruit with the oat bran, oat flakes, toasted buckwheat, yogurt, borage oil, and maple syrup.

Spoon into two bowls and serve.

Wheat contains a protein called gluten, which is difficult to break down, absorb, and assimilate, making it a common food allergen. Women with wheat intolerance are prone to fatigue, depression, bloating, intestinal gas, bowel changes, post-nasal drip, nasal congestion, and frequent colds. Children with wheat intolerance are susceptible to middle ear infections.

Tips:
→ Try pasta made from rice, corn, or buckwheat.
→ Make corn bread rather than whole wheat bread to accompany your meals.
→ Use bread made with rice, millet, or oat flour.
→ Experiment with rice-based crackers topped with tuna, sliced apple, almond butter, or tahini.

Cereal Flakes with Peaches   Serves 2

This warm, peachy mixture is rich in magnesium, which is crucial for our body's cell energy and hormone transportation.

   1 ¼ cups almond or rice milk
   2 tablespoons honey
   1 cup rice flakes
   3 fresh peaches (about 10 ounces)
   1 tablespoon pistachio nuts
   2 tablespoons raisins
   2 tablespoons corn flakes

Heat the milk and honey, stirring, until just before boiling point. Pour the mixture over the rice flakes, cover, and let stand for 10 minutes.

Dip the peaches into boiling water for 20–60 seconds, transfer to a bowl of cold water, then slip off the skins. Pit the peaches and dice the flesh. Chop the pistachios and toast them in a dry nonstick skillet. Gently fold the diced peaches and raisins into the rice flakes.

Sprinkle with the corn flakes and pistachios and serve.

Fruit Salad with Buckwheat and Seeds Serves 2

Grapes contain heart-friendly compounds called flavonoids as well as pterostilbene, a powerful antioxidant.

7 ounces seedless grapes
1 medium apple
$\frac{2}{3}$ cup mango, peeled
2 tablespoons raisins
$\frac{1}{2}$ cup kiwi-strawberry juice
2 ounces buckwheat groats
2 tablespoons sesame seeds
2 tablespoons ground flaxseeds

Wash the fruit. Pluck grapes from stems. Core and cut the apple into eighths, then cut each piece in half. Cut the mango into bite-sized pieces. Place the fruit in a bowl with the raisins and kiwi-strawberry juice.

Toast the buckwheat and seeds in a dry nonstick skillet, tossing occasionally, until you begin to smell them. Cool slightly and sprinkle over the fruit.

Tip: Replace Your Coffee with Green Tea

Green tea, which has been found to fight cancer—thanks to its high concentration of polyphenols. These remarkable compounds have been shown to prevent the formation of cancer-causing compounds, including nitrosamines (formed when the nitrites in cured foods bind with amino acids). They also directly detoxify certain cancer-causing agents.

To avoid the dangers associated with coffee and reap the benefits of green tea, I suggest cutting your coffee consumption in half; for example, if you drink four cups a day, try going down to two cups. You can replace those two cups with two cups of green tea. After two weeks, reduce your coffee intake by half again (from two to one) while still enjoying your two cups of green tea.

Give this another week or so, then eliminate that final cup of coffee. By following this program, you'll be coffee-free and green tea-rich in less than a month!

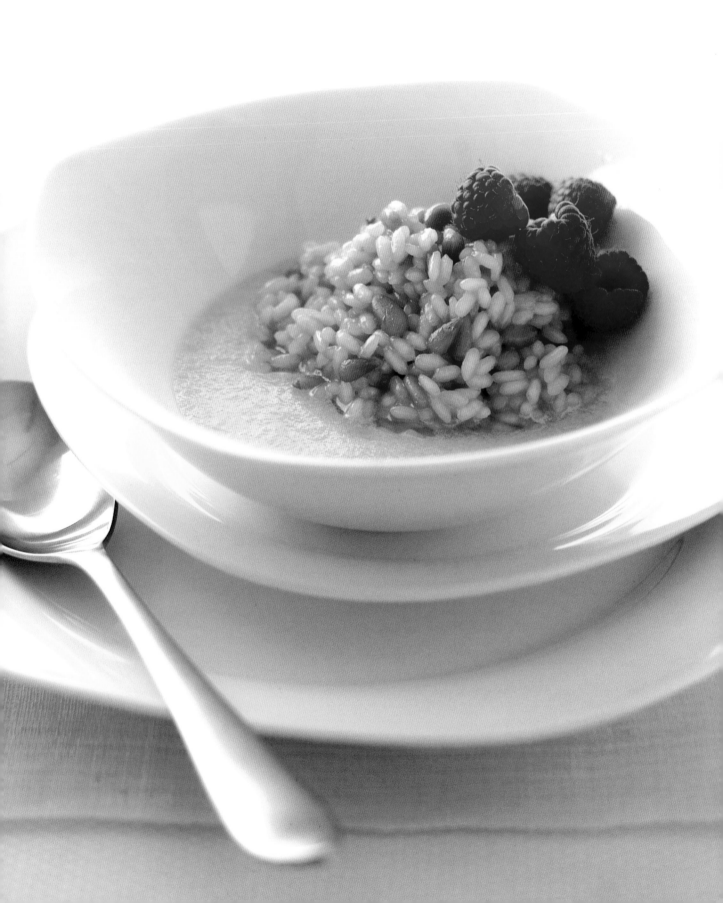

Risotto with Melon Purée and Berries Serves 2

Melons are generally cleansing. They contain carotenoids, which contribute to smooth, healthy skin.

1 teaspoon canola oil
½ cup Arborio rice
2 tablespoons pine nuts
1 ½ cups apple or grape juice
12 ounces cantaloupe, peeled
1 tablespoon honey
1 cup fresh seasonal berries

Heat the oil in a pan over low heat. Add the rice and pine nuts, and sauté until the rice becomes slightly translucent. Pour in half the fruit juice and simmer gently, stirring continuously, until the rice looks chalky, with a white dot in the center of each grain. Add the remaining juice, and bring to a boil again briefly. Remove the pan from heat, cover tightly, and let stand until cool. Refrigerate the mixture until ready to serve, as long as overnight.

Cut the cantaloupe into chunks. In a food processor, purée the cantaloupe chunks with the honey. Wash the berries. Pour the cantaloupe purée into two deep bowls and stir in the berries, portioning evenly.

Top each serving with a scoop of the rice and serve.

Hot Cereal and Flax with Banana Topping Serves 3

The fiber-rich cereal delivers consistent energy through your morning, while the topping gives this breakfast bone-health-boosting potassium. The flax, rich in crucial omega-3 and omega-6 essential fatty acids, promotes proper sugar metabolism and healthy skin.

1 cup buckwheat groats, oats, or quinoa
2–3 cups water (as directed)
1 ½ cups rice or nut milk
2 medium bananas, barely ripe
1 ½ teaspoons vanilla
¼ teaspoon cinnamon
5 tablespoons ground raw flaxseeds

In a heavy saucepan over medium heat, bring the water (per package instructions) to boil. Add grains, reduce heat to simmer, cover, and cook as instructed. Cooking times range according to the grain.

While grains are cooking, combine the milk, bananas, vanilla, and cinnamon in a food processor and blend mixture until smooth.

When cereal is done cooking, remove from heat and let stand a few minutes. Stir in ground flaxseeds, spoon hot cereal into bowls, and top with banana mixture.

Sunshine Muesli Serves 2

Among many sunny ingredients in this eye-opening breakfast, fresh pineapple contains bromelain, a protein-digesting enzyme that aids in digestion, reduces inflammation, and cleanses the skin.

1 ½ cups strawberries
1 small or ¼ large fresh ripe pineapple
2 ounces flaked millet
2 tablespoons oat bran
1 tablespoon bee pollen
½ cup pineapple-orange-guava juice

Gently rinse, hull, and halve the strawberries. Cut off the pineapple rind from the sides, removing as much of the "eyes" as possible. Slice fruit lengthwise into quarters and remove the core. Cut into bite-sized pieces, reserving the juice.

Place the chopped fruit and juice, flaked millet, oat bran, bee pollen, and pineapple-orange-guava juice in a bowl, and mix.

Spoon the muesli into two bowls, and serve.

Waffles with Blueberries Serves 2

Blueberry skins' blue pigment, anthocyanin, protects your cells, revitalizes your body, and keeps you young.

About 3 ounces fresh blueberries
1 teaspoon agave syrup
1 tablespoon dairy-free cream cheese (e.g., Soya Kaas or Tofutti)
2 tablespoons dairy-free yogurt
Black pepper
2 rice-flour or other wheat-free waffles
Fresh thyme leaves

Remove any stems from berries and place in bowl. Crush them lightly with a fork and drizzle with agave syrup.

Blend the cream cheese with the yogurt until smooth, then season with pepper. Fold in the blueberries, then spoon the mixture onto the rice waffles, and garnish with the thyme.

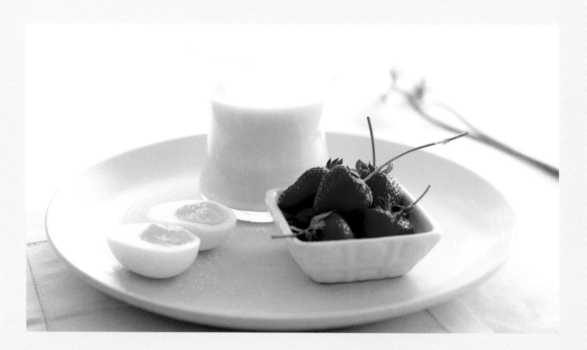

Beautiful Breakfasts

Don't have the time to sit down to hot breakfast? Try some of these easy, healthy, beauty-enhancing breakfast options. All are rich in good fats that keep your hair and skin silky smooth, isoflavones that fend of hot flashes, protein to even your blood sugar levels, and fiber to protect you from heart disease.

→   Hard-boiled egg with mixed berries and a glass of almond milk
→   Soy yogurt with half a banana and ground flaxseed
→   Whip up a fruity concoction from the Shakes & Drinks beauty recipes (see page 31)

Lunch

Broccoli-Sauerkraut Salad Serves 2

Sauerkraut, or fermented cabbage, aids digestion and strengthens tissues. In a 2001 study of dietary habits of postmenopausal Swedish women aged 50–74, those who ate 1–2 servings of Brassica foods (such as cabbage and broccoli) a day had a 20–40 percent lower risk of breast cancer than those who ate virtually none.

5 ounces broccoli florets
1–2 tablespoons water
1 can sweet corn kernels (7 ounces)
8 ounces sauerkraut, drained
2 tablespoons sunflower seeds
1 clove garlic
⅔ cup soy yogurt
2 tablespoons nut oil
1 tablespoon Bragg Liquid Aminos
Sea salt to taste
Black pepper to taste
1 teaspoon fresh thyme leaves
Potato bread or boiled small potatoes for accompaniment

Roughly chop washed broccoli, then purée in a blender or food processor, adding a little water to achieve a smooth texture. Drain the corn. Coarsely chop the sauerkraut with a knife, then mix it well in a bowl with the corn, and puréed broccoli. Coarsely chop the sunflower seeds. Peel and finely chop the garlic.

To make the dressing, whisk the sunflower seeds, garlic, soy yogurt, oil, and Bragg Liquid Aminos in a bowl until mixed well. Season with the salt, pepper, and thyme. Toss the vegetables with the dressing, arrange on plates, and serve with bread or potatoes.

Chopped Egg and Tuna Sandwich Serves 2

Not the villains they once were thought to be, eggs pack protein, brain-nurturing choline, and antioxidant-rich carotenoids.

- 1 hard-boiled egg, peeled
- 1 can water-packed tuna (6 ounces)
- 3 tablespoons olive oil
- 1 tablespoon fresh lemon juice
- 2 tablespoons capers
- Black pepper to taste
- Worcestershire sauce to taste
- 2 whole-grain, wheat-free rolls (i.e., made from amaranth, buckwheat, oat, or spelt flour)
- 2–3 leaves radicchio

Separate the yolk from the egg, chop the white, and set aside. In a food processor, blend the drained tuna, oil, the egg yolk, and lemon juice to a paste. Transfer mixture to a bowl and stir in capers, pepper, and Worcestershire.

Split the rolls and spread with the tuna paste. Cut washed and dried radicchio into strips, and arrange on the rolls. Sprinkle the egg white over the open-faced sandwiches.

Mediterranean Zucchini Serves 4

Besides boasting a wide variety of female-beneficial nutrients, including potassium and phosphorus, this marinated zucchini makes the perfect lunch accompanied by a wheat-free crusty bread spread with hummus or dairy-free cream cheese.

2–3 medium-small zucchini (about 1 pound)
2 tablespoons olive oil
1 ½–2 teaspoons minced garlic (about 4 cloves)
1 tablespoon fresh basil, mint, or thyme
1 tablespoon Bragg Liquid Aminos
Dash of salt

Wash and dry zucchini; slice diagonally into long ⅓-inch-thick ovals. Coat the bottom of a large, heavy skillet with oil and heat. Sauté zucchini ovals until gold freckles appear on both sides and centers are tender. Drain on paper towels. Lower the heat and sauté the garlic until just golden, stirring constantly.

Rinse, shake dry, and chop the fresh herbs. On a platter or in a bowl, sprinkle the zucchini with the chopped herbs, Bragg Liquid Aminos, salt, and garlic. Cover and marinate; serve at room temperature.

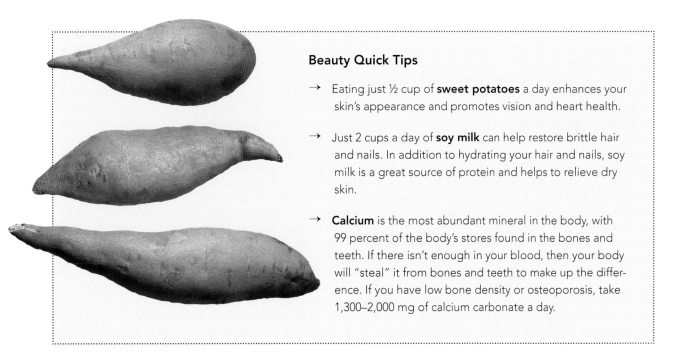

Beauty Quick Tips

→ Eating just ½ cup of **sweet potatoes** a day enhances your skin's appearance and promotes vision and heart health.

→ Just 2 cups a day of **soy milk** can help restore brittle hair and nails. In addition to hydrating your hair and nails, soy milk is a great source of protein and helps to relieve dry skin.

→ **Calcium** is the most abundant mineral in the body, with 99 percent of the body's stores found in the bones and teeth. If there isn't enough in your blood, then your body will "steal" it from bones and teeth to make up the difference. If you have low bone density or osteoporosis, take 1,300–2,000 mg of calcium carbonate a day.

Pumpkin Cream Soup Serves 2

Not just for Halloween carvings, pumpkin is rich in vitamin A, which plays a part in smooth, healthy skin.

24 ounces pumpkin, canned or roughly chopped, if fresh
1 onion
1 tablespoon olive oil
Salt to taste
Pepper to taste
1 cup carrot juice
2 tablespoons plain non-dairy yogurt
Allspice to taste
Fresh lemon juice to taste
1 ounce dried currants
½ ounce pumpkin seeds, roughly chopped

Roughly chop pumpkin flesh if using fresh. Peel and finely chop the onion. If using fresh pumpkin, add it and onion to a saucepan with the oil, season with salt and pepper, and sauté over medium heat until tender. If using canned pumpkin, add it now to sautéed onion and purée with carrot juice and yogurt.

Season with the allspice and lemon juice. Add the currants and pumpkin seeds, heat through, and serve.

Red Lentils With Carrot-Spinach Confetti Serves 2

Vitamin C-rich grapefruit stimulates the circulatory system, contributing to radiant skin.

2 tablespoons dried seaweed (i.e., arame or dulce)
1 ½ cups water
¾ cup red lentils
Sea salt to taste
½ teaspoon allspice
7 ounces baby carrots
7 ounces spinach leaves (from a pre-washed, bagged spinach salad)
1 small onion
1 tablespoon pink grapefruit juice
1 teaspoon pink grapefruit zest
3 tablespoons nut or avocado oil
1 teaspoon dry mustard
Black pepper to taste
Hot steamed brown rice for accompaniment

In a saucepan, soak the sea vegetables in the water for 5 minutes. Add the lentils, salt, and allspice. Simmer covered over low heat for 10 minutes; remove from the heat to prevent the seaweed from absorbing too much liquid.

Meanwhile, coarsely grate the carrots. Cut the spinach leaves into strips. Peel and finely chop the onion. Add the grapefruit juice, zest, oil, and dry mustard to the lentil and sea vegetables mixture, and carefully stir in the grated carrot and spinach strips. Season with salt and pepper, and serve warm with the rice.

Salmon-Watercress Sandwich Serves 2

A magnificent supply of omega-3s, salmon is also an excellent source of selenium and a very good source of protein, niacin, and vitamin B12.

2 whole-grain, wheat-free rolls (i.e., made from amaranth, buckwheat, oat, or spelt flour)
1 bunch watercress
¼ cup plain, non-dairy yogurt
1 teaspoon flaxseed oil
Sea salt to taste
Black pepper to taste
1 teaspoon fresh lemon juice
4 slices smoked salmon

Halve the rolls. Rinse the watercress under cold, running water, and scissor off the leaves, reserving some for garnish. Mix the watercress with the yogurt, oil, salt, pepper, and lemon juice, and spread on the halved rolls.

Top with the smoked salmon in even portions, and garnish with the remaining watercress.

Smoked Salmon Salad Serves 2

Mustard helps with digestion, has anti-inflammatory effects, and promotes blood flow to your body's tissues.

2 tablespoons pumpkin seed oil
1 tablespoon avocado oil
1 tablespoon orange juice
7 tablespoons pineapple juice
Sea salt to taste
Black pepper to taste
1 teaspoon dry mustard
4 ounces arugula
6 ounces smoked salmon, very thinly sliced
2 tablespoons pumpkin seeds
Wheat-free ciabatta bread or baguette for accompaniment

For the dressing, mix the oils, juices, salt, pepper, and mustard in a bowl, and whisk well.

Wash and shake dry the arugula. Set aside half the arugula, divide the rest among two plates, and drizzle with a little dressing. Then, arrange the salmon and remaining arugula leaves on top and drizzle with the remaining dressing. Coarsely chop the pumpkin seeds and sprinkle over the salad. Let salads stand for about 30 minutes to blend the flavors.

Fresh bread makes a nice accompaniment.

Tip: Invest in a Couple of Digestive Aids

Plant-derived enzymes such as bromelain and pancreatin go a long way to counteracting the effects of immoderate eating and drinking. Just 500–1,000 mg of bromelain a day can reduce the pain, gas, and bowel frequency associated with poor digestion. A daily dosage of 300–500 mg of pancreatin helps fight pain and gas by promoting better digestion and uptake of nutrients in your digestive tract

Stuffed Tomatoes Serves 2

Tomatoes contain beneficial amounts of potassium, magnesium, and the antioxidant lycopene.

6 medium tomatoes (about 1 pound)
Salt and pepper to taste
½ cup buckwheat groats
2–3 green onions
1 clove garlic
8 ounces sauerkraut, drained
1 bunch fresh dill
1 tablespoon fresh lemon juice
2 tablespoons nut or avocado oil

Thinly slice off the tops (for use as lids) of washed tomatoes, and scoop out the insides with a spoon; reserve the tomato pulp for another use. Put the tomatoes upside down in sieve to drain. Then season tomato cavities with salt and pepper.

Lightly toast the buckwheat groats in a nonstick skillet. Thinly slice the washed green onions. Peel and finely chop the garlic. Slice the sauerkraut into fine slivers. Wash the dill and remove feathery leaves from stalks.

In a bowl, combine the buckwheat, green onions, garlic, sauerkraut, and dill. Add the salt, pepper, lemon juice, and oil and mix carefully. Season the stuffing well and evenly portion into the tomatoes. Replace the tomatoes' "lids," arrange on plates, and serve.

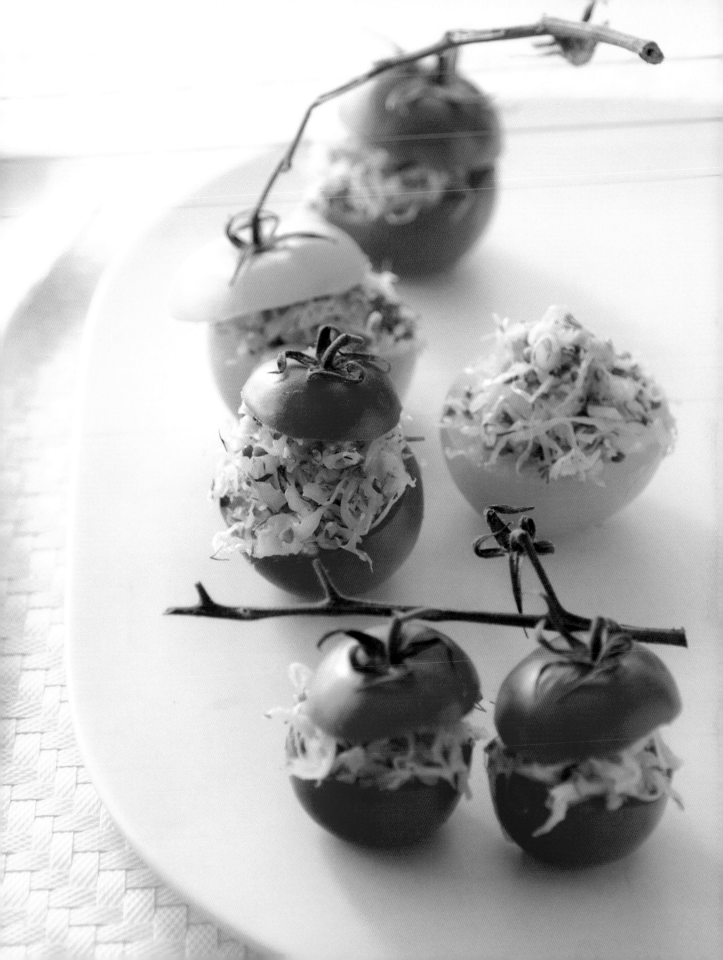

Dinner

Amaranth-Vegetable Stir-Fry Serves 2

Revered by the Aztecs as a giver of strength, amaranth is high in protein and is less acid-forming than many other grains.

½ cup amaranth
1 teaspoon dried lemon grass
1 cup vegetable stock
2 green onions
10 ounces baby carrots
5 ounces celery
7 ounces mushrooms
2 tablespoons corn oil
2 ounces skinned almonds
4 ounces bean sprouts
1 tablespoon sesame oil
Soy sauce to taste

Boil the amaranth, lemon grass, and stock together in a saucepan. Reduce the heat and simmer the amaranth for 15 minutes. Trim the washed green onions and slice thinly. Peel the washed carrots and slice into ¼-inch-thick coins. Wash and trim the celery and cut into 1-inch matchsticks. Rinse and wipe the mushrooms clean and, depending on size, chop them into four or eight pieces.

Heat the corn oil in a wok or large skillet over medium heat and stir-fry the almonds until their aroma is evident. Add the carrots and stir-fry briefly. Add the celery, mushrooms, green onions, and bean sprouts and stir-fry for 5 minutes. Add the cooked amaranth and the sesame oil, and stir-fry for a moment and add the soy sauce. Remove the lemon grass and serve immediately.

Chicken Stir-Fry with Avocado Serves 2

Loaded with unsaturated fatty acids, avocadoes promote soft skin, healthy cell walls, and strong nerves.

1 tablespoon fresh lemon juice
Sea salt to taste
Black pepper to taste
Paprika
½ teaspoon ground star anise
7 ounces chicken breast
1 green bell pepper
2 cloves garlic
1 onion
1–2 tablespoons olive oil
1 bunch fresh Italian parsley
1 avocado
10 black olives, pitted
Steamed millet or brown rice for accompaniment

Combine the lemon juice, salt, pepper, a pinch of paprika, and the star anise in a shallow bowl. Slice the chicken into thin strips, and add the chicken to the bowl, turning to coat.

Remove the stem, ribs, and seeds from the bell pepper, rinse, and coarsely chop. Peel and finely chop the garlic and onion.

Drain the chicken. In a wok or large skillet, heat the oil over medium-high heat, add the chicken, and brown on all sides. Add a pinch of paprika, the garlic and onion, and stir-fry for 5 minutes. Wash and shake dry the parsley, remove the leaves from the stems, and chop. Halve the avocado, remove the pit, and with a paring knife, score the flesh within the skin, then scoop out flesh with a spoon. Mix the avocado, olives and parsley, and season to taste with lemon juice, salt, and pepper.

Divide the chicken mixture among serving dishes, top with the avocado mixture, and serve with the millet or rice.

Boiled Potatoes with Creamy Sauce Serves 2

With loads of valuable plant protein and vitamins C and B6, these alkaline-forming tubers are new cell builders.

1 pound small red-skinned potatoes
Sea salt to taste
1 small red bell pepper
1 shallot
1 clove garlic
1 bunch fresh Italian parsley
8 ounces dairy-free cream cheese (e.g., Soya Kaas or Tofutti)
1 tablespoon oat bran
1 tablespoon yeast flakes
1 tablespoon flaxseed oil
Tabasco sauce to taste
About ½ cup spring water

Cover the washed potatoes with salted water in a saucepan. Cover the pan with a lid and bring the water to a boil for about 20 minutes, until tender.

Meanwhile, remove the stem, ribs, and seeds from the bell pepper, rinse, and cut into small squares. Peel and dice the shallot and garlic. Wash and shake dry the parsley, and finely chop the leaves. Place the cream cheese in a bowl and mix with the parsley, oat bran, yeast flakes, flaxseed oil, Tabasco, and enough water to make a smooth sauce. Mix in the chopped bell pepper, the diced shallot, and the garlic. Season and serve with the warm, drained potatoes.

Fish Stew Serves 2

Bright red radicchio stimulates digestion, is soothing, and cleanses the blood.

10 ounces mild white fish fillets
1 tablespoon cider vinegar
Sea salt to taste
1 leek
10 prunes, pitted
1 tablespoon canola oil
2 ½ cups fish or vegetable stock
1 bay leaf
3 peppercorns
2 whole clove
⅔ cup French green lentils
1 head radicchio
1 teaspoon honey
Wheat-free baguette for accompaniment

Wash and pat dry the fish fillets, drizzle with cider vinegar, and season with salt. Trim off the leek's root and dark green leaves and halve it lengthwise. Wash it well and cut into thin slices. Quarter the prunes lengthwise.

In a skillet, heat the oil over medium heat. Add the leek and sauté until glazed. Add the stock, salt, bay leaf, peppercorns, cloves, prunes, and lentils. Cover tightly and simmer over low heat for about 8 minutes; the lentils will retain some firmness.

Trim and wash the radicchio, and slice the leaves into strips. Add the radicchio and the fish, with the vinegar marinade, to the lentils, and simmer gently for another 3–4 minutes over low heat. Stir in the honey and season with salt.

Arrange on plates and serve with the baguette.

New England-Style Chowder Serves 4

The selenium, vitamin D, and omega-3 fats found in wild-caught cod have anti-inflammatory effects, while high-fiber corn promotes cardiovascular health, memory maintenance, and energy production, even under stress.

- 3 tablespoons shredded carrot
- 2 tablespoons diced celery
- 2 tablespoons minced fresh onion
- 2 cups diced, peeled baking potato (about ½ pound)
- 2 tablespoons olive oil
- 3 tablespoons oat or rice flour
- 3 ½ cups rice or nut milk
- ½ teaspoon miso
- ¼ teaspoon pepper
- 16 ounces wild cod fillets
- 1 cup corn

Wash, trim, and shred the carrot. Rinse and dice the celery, peel and mince the onion, and peel and dice the potatoes.

Heat olive oil in a saucepan over medium heat. Add carrot, celery, and onion; sauté 2 minutes. Stir in flour; gradually add 2 ½ cups milk, stirring constantly with a whisk. Add potato, miso, and pepper; bring to a boil. Reduce heat. Simmer, uncovered, 30 minutes; stir occasionally.

Meanwhile, rinse and cut cod into 1-inch pieces. Add fish, corn, and remaining 1 cup milk to chowder; cook an additional 10 minutes or until fish is done.

Niçoise Salad Serves 2

Also lovely with salmon, this supper salad is packed with hair-healthy nutrients.

    2 grilled fresh tuna steaks (about 4 ounces each)
    2 cups mixed lettuce greens (e.g., romaine, arugula, and red leaf)
    1 cup trimmed watercress (about ¼ bunch)
    ¼ cup garbanzo beans
    2 tablespoons olive oil
    1 teaspoon Bragg Liquid Aminos
    ½ pound small red potatoes
    ½ pound fresh green beans
    2 hard-boiled eggs
    10–20 small black olives, pitted

Slice tuna steaks into ½-inch slices. Wash and shake dry the greens and watercress. Place greens, watercress, and garbanzos in a large bowl. Toss with 1 tablespoon olive oil and ½ teaspoon Bragg Liquid Aminos. Portion the dressed lettuce onto two large plates.

Steam potatoes, covered, 3 minutes. Add green beans, and steam, covered, an additional 8 minutes or until vegetables are crisp-tender; cool.

Slice the hard-boiled eggs. Toss green beans and sliced eggs with remaining 1 tablespoon olive oil and ½ teaspoon Bragg Liquid Aminos.

Place potatoes around outer rim of plates and green beans in the center. Coarsely chop the pitted olives. Top salads with tuna slices and olives.

Stir-Fried Halibut with Vegetables Serves 2

Sea vegetables are bursting with nutrients, including calcium, iodine, iron, and vitamin B12.

2 tablespoons dried seaweed (e.g., arame or dulce)
½ cup plus 2 tablespoons water
10 ounces halibut steak
Walnut-sized piece of fresh ginger
1 teaspoon dry mustard
1 tablespoon tamari, plus more to taste
1 tablespoon fresh lemon juice
1 leek
7 ounces carrots
7 ounces celery
5 ounces sugar snap peas or green beans
1 teaspoon canola oil
Sea salt to taste
Black pepper to taste
Soy sauce to taste
1 tablespoon sesame oil
Cooked potatoes, wild rice, or millet

Soak the seaweed in ½ cup water for 5 minutes. Rinse, pat dry, and cube the halibut. Peel and mince the ginger, then mix it with the dry mustard, tamari, lemon juice, and the 2 tablespoons water. Brush the mustard mixture over the fish. Wash and trim the remaining vegetables. Trim off the leek's root and dark green leaves, halve it lengthwise, and cut into fine rings. Peel the carrots and cut into matchsticks. Chop the celery crosswise into bite-sized pieces. Discard the stalks from the sugar snap peas or beans, and remove any strings. Drain the seaweed well.

Heat the canola oil in a nonstick skillet over medium-high heat, and brown the fish on both sides. Add the leek, carrots, celery, peas or beans, and the seaweed. Season with salt and pepper, and stir-fry for about 5–7 minutes, until the fish and vegetables are cooked through. Season with soy sauce and stir in the sesame oil.

Serve with potatoes, wild rice, or millet.

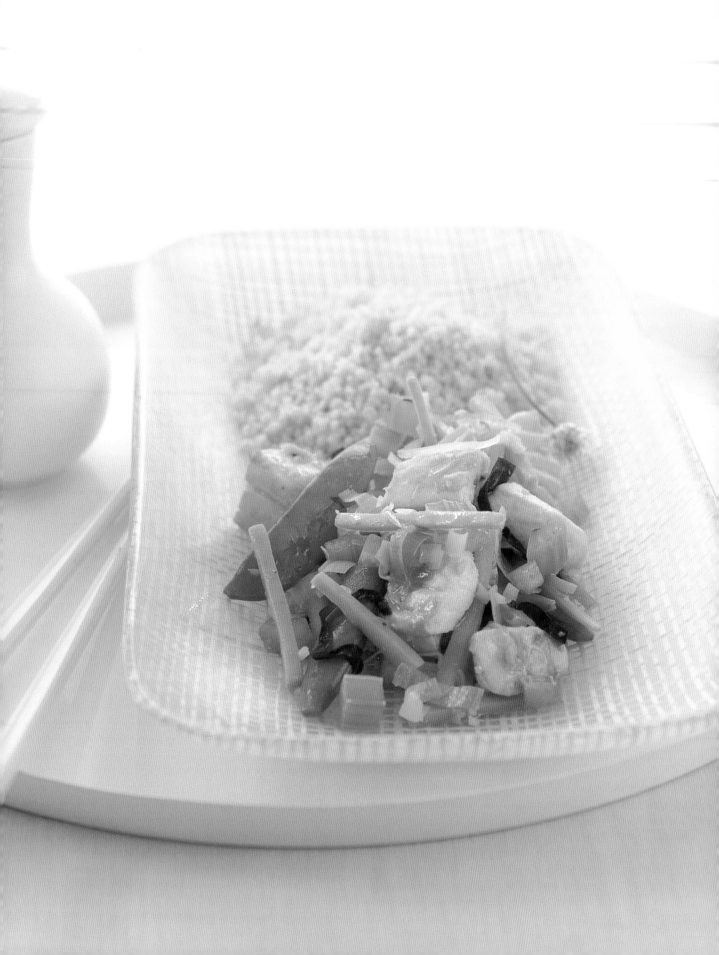

Turkey and Endive Sauté   Serves 2

Endive stimulates the stomach, spleen, liver, and gall bladder.

7 ounces boneless turkey breast
Sea salt to taste
Black pepper to taste
Sweet paprika to taste
2 heads Belgian endive
1 teaspoon canola oil
½ can diced carrots (about 14.5 ounces)
1 clove garlic
4 ounces bean sprouts
1 tablespoon sesame oil
4 ounces mozzarella soy cheese
Wheat-free baguette for accompaniment

Carve the turkey breast against the grain into ½-inch slices. Season with salt, pepper, and paprika. Trim the washed endive and halve it lengthwise.

In a saucepan, sauté the endive in canola oil over medium-high heat until just brown at the edges. Add the turkey and brown on all sides. Add the carrots. Cover tightly and simmer gently for 5 minutes over low heat. Peel the garlic and slice thinly. Add it with the bean sprouts and sesame oil to the skillet.

Drain the soy mozzarella, cut into slices, and place on the endive. Simmer gently over low heat until the cheese melts. Arrange on plates and serve with the baguette.

Desserts

Banana "Ice Cream" Serves 4

Not only is this a cold, sweet, and creamy treat, but bananas are a source of the magnesium and potassium you need to keep your heart muscle healthy.

4 large well-ripened bananas

Peel and slice bananas into ½-inch-thick medallions. Put slices on a baking sheet or wax-paper-lined plate large enough to freeze bananas in a single layer. Freeze for 1 hour or as long as two days uncovered.

Purée the frozen slices in a food processor or blender. Stop the machine to scrape container sides. Continue blending until the thawing bananas become smooth and creamy. Serve immediately.

Note: Frozen banana slices will keep for several weeks in a covered container or freezer bag.

Blackberry Sorbet Float Serves 2

Berries are veritable fonts of fiber; antioxidants; the vitamins A, C, E, and folic acid; and the minerals potassium and calcium.

9 ounces fresh blackberries
Scant ½ cup maple syrup
Pinch of ground cinnamon
Sparkling water

Swish the blackberries in water, then drain, and gently pat dry. Purée the berries and press through the sieve into a freezer-proof bowl. Stir in the maple syrup. Place the mixture in the freezer, stirring every 30 minutes, until frozen. Transfer the sorbet to the refrigerator about 30 minutes before serving.

Stir the sorbet well, evenly spoon it into two glasses, sprinkle with cinnamon, and top with sparkling water.

See page 74 for photo of Blackberry Sorbet Float.

Chocolate Pudding Serves 2

Dates offer a sweet dose of high fiber with plenty of iron and potassium. Find anti-oxidant- and polyphenol-rich organic cocoa in most Whole Foods stores, many organic markets, or www.healthyshopping.com.

8 dried dates, pitted
2 ½ cups almond milk
5 tablespoons Dagoba or other high-quality, organic cocoa powder
2 tablespoons cornstarch
2 tablespoons water

If your dried dates are hard, steam them briefly until softened. Purée moist dates in a blender or food processor. Transfer purée to a saucepan, and gradually whisk in the milk and cocoa powder. Bring to a boil, stirring constantly. Mix the cornstarch with the water, stir this into the cocoa mixture, and simmer gently for 1 minute over low heat.

Spoon evenly into two dessert bowls and chill until ready to serve.

Sugar is a major source of dietary acid. When it is processed, all the vitamins and minerals are removed; what remains is simple sugar, glucose, which breaks down rapidly in your digestive system producing acids. Sugar also makes your liver work harder to produce bile and other essential digestive enzymes. Refined sugar may also:

→   Contribute to blood sugar imbalances;
→   Increase perimenopausal anxiety, irritability, and nervous tension;
→   Deplete B-complex vitamins and minerals;
→   Intensify fatigue; and
→   Feed *Candida* fungus, leading to yeast infections.

Fresh Fruit Kabobs   Serves 8

The fruit on these skewers are all fabulously effective detoxifiers to drive healthy skin. Serve as a snack or dessert.

  8 bamboo skewers (9-inches long)
  ½ cup mango chunks, cut into 1-inch chunks
  ½ cup cantaloupe chunks, cut into 1-inch chunks
  ½ cup pineapple chunks, cut into 1-inch chunks
  1 small bunch red seedless grapes
  2 cups mango-, pineapple-, or vanilla-flavored soy or other dairy-free yogurt

On each skewer alternate mango sections with cantaloupe and pineapple chunks. Place a grape on each end of each skewer. Arrange kabobs on a platter with yogurt as dip.

Maplenut Sundae   Serves 4–6

Heart-healthy walnuts are known as brain food for their high concentration of omega-3 fats.

  ¾ cup walnut pieces
  ½ cup maple syrup
  Dairy-free frozen yogurt or ice cream

Toast raw walnut pieces in a single layer on an ungreased tray in a 350° F oven for about 5 minutes, until they're fragrant and lightly browned.

Combine the toasted nuts with the maple syrup. Warm mixture if you like. Spoon over frozen yogurt or ice cream.

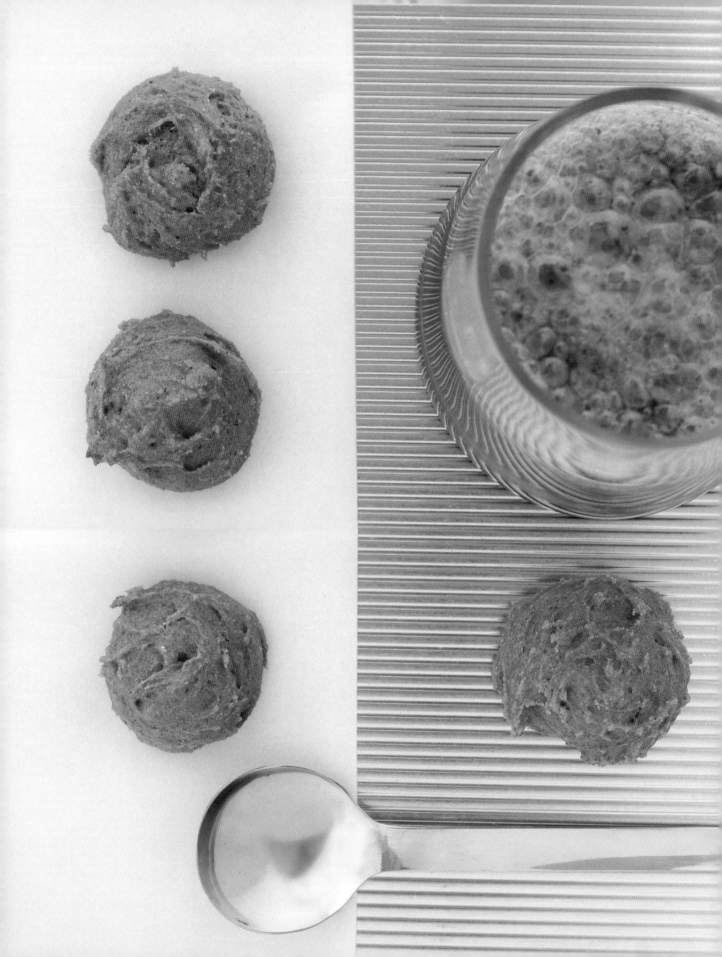

Pumpkin Cookies Makes 2 dozen

Pumpkin is loaded with skin-protecting vitamin A. Xylitol is a little-known plant sugar that won't raise your blood sugar as fast as regular sugar, and it raises the pH in the mouth so it helps prevent dental cavities. It even has one-third fewer calories than regular sugar.

1 cup quinoa flour
1 cup spelt or kamut flour
½ teaspoon baking soda
1 teaspoon cinnamon
½ teaspoon ginger
¼ teaspoon nutmeg
¼ teaspoon allspice
¾ cup puréed, cooked pumpkin
¾ cup xylitol
½ cup plain dairy-free yogurt
2 tablespoons cold-pressed vegetable oil

Preheat oven to 350°F.

Mix flours, soda, cinnamon, ginger, nutmeg, and allspice in a mixing bowl; set aside. Stir together pumpkin, xylitol, yogurt, and oil in another bowl. Add wet to dry ingredients and stir until combined.

Lightly oil a cookie sheet and drop by tablespoons onto cookie sheet. Bake 15 minutes. If frosting, cool cookies first on a rack then frost tops.

See page 71 for the Blackberry Sorbet Float, also featured on the opposite page.

Plum Dumplings   Serves 2

Plums boost iron absorption into the body, contain loads of collagen-building vitamin C, and boast high levels of antioxidant protection from phytonutrients called phenols.

  1 pound baking potatoes
  Salt to taste
  3 tablespoons oat, spelt, or rice flour
  2–3 tablespoons potato flour
  14 ounces small fresh plums
  1 teaspoon ground cinnamon
  2 tablespoons water
  4 tablespoons maple syrup
  2 tablespoons nut oil
  2 tablespoons finely chopped hazelnuts

Wash the potatoes and steam them until tender, about 20–30 minutes. Peel the potatoes while still hot and push them through a potato ricer. Let stand for a few minutes until steam abates. Stir into the riced potatoes a pinch of salt, the flour, and enough potato flour to bind the mixture but keep it very soft.

Wash the plums. Select 12 and dry them. Carefully remove the stones and push the plum halves together so that they appear to be intact. Divide the dough into 12 equal pieces, press a plum into the center of each piece, and gently roll into a ball. Halve the remaining plums, remove the stones, and gently simmer the plums with ½ teaspoon of the cinnamon and the water until tender. Into the compote, stir 2 tablespoons of the maple syrup and chill.

In a 4-quart saucepan, bring 2 ½–3 quarts salted water to a boil. Submerge dumplings in the water and simmer, uncovered, for 10 minutes, until they rise to the top. Remove with a slotted spoon and drain.

In a skillet, heat the oil over medium heat and sauté the nuts until golden. Add the remaining ½ teaspoon cinnamon and toss the plum dumplings into this mixture to coat. Drizzle dumplings with the remaining 2 tablespoons of syrup and serve with the compote.

Yum Yam Frosting   Makes ¾–1 cup (enough to frost 2 dozen cookies or 1-layer cake)

This yammy recipe is high in beta-carotene, which helps boost your immune system, improves the health of your skin, suppresses premenstrual acne and oily skin, and balances the adrenal system to enhance energy and stamina.

1 cup mashed baked yams
2 ounces or ¼ cup softened dairy-free cream cheese or soft tofu
2 teaspoons canola oil
2 tablespoons maple syrup
1 teaspoon orange juice

Place yams, cream cheese, oil, syrup, and juice in a bowl and cream together. Purée in a food processor or with a hand mixer until smooth and spreadable.

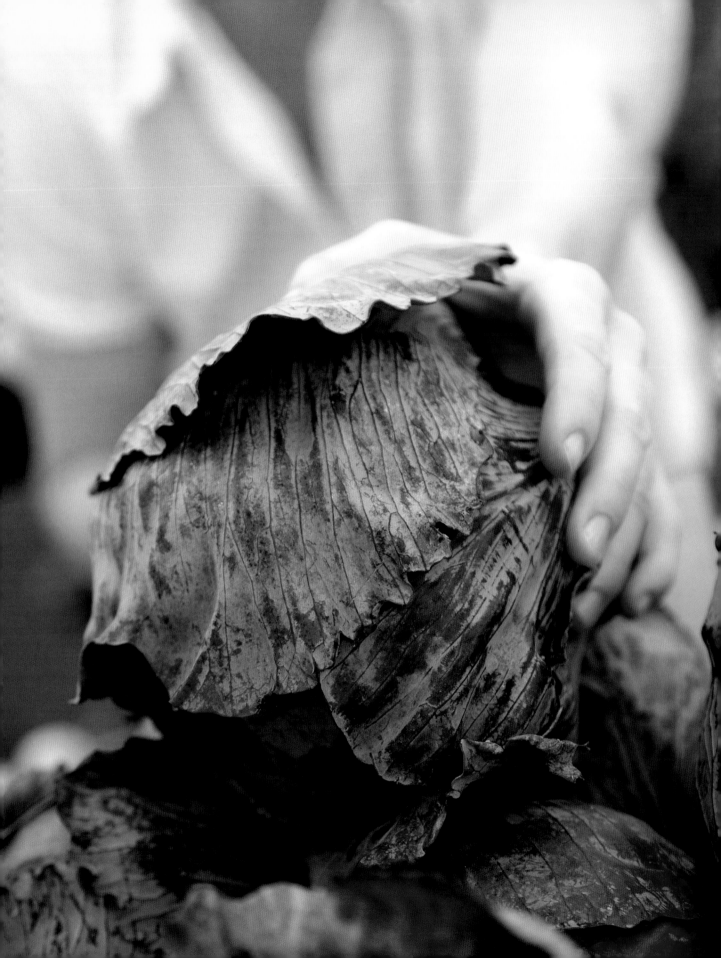

Natural Weight Loss

In my practice, I've seen many frustrated overweight women who have starved themselves, tried every diet on the market, and exercised regularly—sometimes intensely—in an attempt to lose the weight they put on as they aged. Some lost weight for a while, but once they returned to so-called "normal" eating, the pounds returned. One friend even joked that she had lost over 100 pounds—but it was the same ten pounds over and over again!

If this sounds familiar, you might be asking, why you gained weight, how it could have been prevented, and whether there is any way to shed it now. The hardline answer from conventional medicine is, you gained the weight because you ate too many calories, you could have prevented it by eating less, and how to shed it now should be obvious: EAT LESS. That's not only unhelpful, it's simply not true.

I have seen that, for most women, the inability to maintain their optimal weight is due not only to the number of calories they are consuming, but also to the influence of various chemical and physiological imbalances that make weight loss much more difficult and frustrating. This is why I don't put women on a one-size-fits-all diet. To me, that implies a short-term fix, and it just plain doesn't work. What most women need is a long-term solution they can live with. The only real way to lose those excess pounds and maintain your optimal weight over the long haul is with a health and lifestyle overhaul. That's what I'm going to give you in this chapter. Let's talk about the physiology of my program first, so you understand why it works so well. Then, I'll touch on the role stress plays and why exercise is so important. Finally, I'll turn you loose with recipes that'll get you firmly and deliciously on the path to your optimal body weight.

Rebalance Your Body

It is essential that you assess the role that chemical imbalances play in causing your excess weight. Chemical imbalances not only cause weight gain, they are responsible for many other uncomfortable physical and emotional symptoms as well. A partial list of the chemical imbalances that can lead to weight gain include thyroid dysfunction, estrogen dominance, insulin resistance, slowing of the metabolism, food allergies (which can cause the accumulation of inflammatory fluids, or "false fat"), and imbalances in brain chemistry that cause mood disturbances, such as depression. Very often, a woman is unknowingly struggling with several of these imbalances, which seem to feed into each other. That's because in many ways, they are all branches of the same "weed" that's growing from a "soil" that's excessively acidic. Correct that acidity, and suddenly all those imbalances become less entrenched. In fact, once a woman has restored an optimal pH, what commonly happens is that one chemical imbalance reveals itself as the "main" one, and with some targeted attention to that problem, all the others start resolving themselves.

Eliminate False Fat

After years of clinical practice treating thousands of patients, I've learned that, for many women, weight gain is related to the accumulation of not only "real" fat but also "false fat." We store excess "real" fat when we either consume too many calories or are unable to burn them efficiently. Chemical imbalances, improper diet, eating for unresolved emotional issues, and a sedentary lifestyle all can contribute to this.

In contrast, "false fat" is due to the accumulation of excess fluids, which we experience as bloating and swelling. This is the result of inflammation, a process that occurs when tissue is damaged or injured. The fact is all traumatic injuries produce an inflammatory response. However, inflammation can occur as a result of stressors, as well—infectious bacteria, viruses, allergens, toxins. No matter where, or how, the injury occurs, the physiologic result is the same—redness, swelling, bloating, pain, stiffness, and a reduced range of motion. The swelling and bloating are the result of the tissues being infiltrated with inflammatory fluid. This is where "false fat" comes in.

Your intestinal tract is a large organ, and it normally takes up a lot of space in your abdomen. When it's been injured, all those lengths of "tubing" are bloated, which can result in astonishing enlargement of the abdomen. The inflammatory response also causes swelling in the skin and subcutaneous fat, including the wall of your abdomen. The result is an even bigger tummy, as well as puffiness of the upper body, face, and extremities. You can see why no amount of "dieting," and no amount of crunches, is going to flatten a midriff that's bloated in this way, because reduced calories and sit-ups aren't addressing the real problem. It'd be like fighting a house fire by washing your car.

That's why a successful weight loss program must start with eliminating the cause of false fat. And, as much as you'd love to drop a couple dress sizes, there's actually another, even more important reason to eliminate false fat—the inflammation that causes it is also seriously affecting your health. Recurrent colds, sinusitis, bronchitis, urinary tract infections, allergies, rheumatoid arthritis, asthma, colitis, endometriosis, and even heart disease, all have been linked to inflammation within your blood vessels. Not only will putting out the inflammatory fire within your body make it easier for you to lose excess inches, but it will improve your overall state of health. And the most effective way to throw water on that fire is to replace common, inflammation-causing foods with healthy substitutes, and take natural anti-inflammatory nutritional supplements.

Foods that Trigger False Fat

Certain foods can trigger inflammation, thereby causing false fat, through three mechanisms: allergic reactions; liver injury; and production of series-2 prostaglandins. When your body detects an allergen, it releases inflammatory histamines and other fiery chemicals to the affected areas. Because food allergies most frequently affect the intestines, the result is bloating and fluid retention in the abdomen. Enzyme deficiency is the most likely culprit for developing these food allergies in the first place. As you age, your production of anti-inflammatory digestive enzymes diminishes, creating a greater likelihood of developing allergic reactions to various foods. For example, I have had many patients suddenly become intolerant of wheat or dairy products when they reach their forties and fifties.

Common Food Allergens

Wheat	Dairy products
Rye	Corn
Soy	Chocolate
Tomatoes	Citrus fruits
Strawberries	Nuts
Pork	Shellfish
Eggs	

Foods can also injure your liver. When your liver function is impaired and cannot fully perform its duties of detoxification, toxins accumulate in your body. Alcohol, red meat, dairy products, and some nuts, as well as foods that are deep fried or high in refined sugar, are especially difficult for your liver to process. Alcohol is particularly taxing and can significantly diminish your liver's ability to operate at peak performance. In fact, chronic overconsumption of alcohol can cause inflammatory changes within the liver itself, leading to fibrosis and permanent damage to the liver's cells. Increased alcohol consumption can also cause mild inflammation of the pancreas. The result: More abdominal bloating, swelling, and discomfort. Similarly, excess sugar consumption can stun the liver. When your liver stores too much glucose, it must work harder to produce bile and essential digestive enzymes. Over time, this all takes a tremendous toll on the liver, resulting in damage to the liver cells, which in turns manifests as even more inflammation.

Prostaglandins, short-lived hormones produced within your body, can be either inflammatory (series-2) or anti-inflammatory (series-1 and series-3). Your body converts dietary essential fatty acids (EFAs) into prostaglandins, and the type of prostaglandins you produce depends upon the type of fats you consume. Simply increasing your consumption of foods from the series-1 and series-3 category (omega-3 EFAs, which are rich in such foods as cold-water fish, flaxseeds, soybeans, and walnuts), and cutting down on foods in the inflammatory series-2 category, such as red meat and animal fat sources like poultry skin, will help to eliminate this kind of false fat. Also, because too few protective omega-3s can also increase your tendency towards inflammation, I recommend taking one to two tablespoons of flaxseed oil each day. I like to include it in my freshly mixed salad dressings, or whirl it into my daily smoothie.

Substituting Foods to Avoid False Fat

If dietary inflammation is a source of false fat for you, it is crucial that you pinpoint the specific culprits that apply to you, then eliminate or minimize your intake of them, replacing them with healthier, anti-inflammatory choices.

To help you do the detective work, I recommend keeping a food diary. Some of my patients keep their diaries in a notebook, others simply list their daily intake on Post It's stuck to the fridge. Most likely, you'll find that the offending foods are those you either crave or eat all the time. You may also want to consult a complementary physician who can help you evaluate this issue. You can call the American College for the Advancement of Medicine (ACAM) at 888.439.6891 or log onto *www.healthfinder.gov/orgs* to locate a physician near you.

There are wonderful and tasty substitutes now available for the foods you decide to eliminate. I have never had patients eliminate foods without adding a substitute that they were happy with. I have made many food substitutions myself, especially when recreating a recipe from a standard cookbook or one of those rich and delicious selections from *Gourmet* or *Bon Appetit* magazine. For a list of suggested food substitutions, see page 18 or log onto my Web site at *www.drlark.com*.

Natural Anti-Inflammatories

There are a number of natural anti-inflammatories that can be used to help prevent false fat. In particular, I recommend digestive enzymes, methylsulfonylmethane (MSM), quercetin, and buffered vitamin C.

Pancreatic digestive enzymes are one of your body's most important ways of not only digesting food, but also breaking up inflammation, regardless of its source or location. To supplement your body's own production of digestive enzymes, eat pineapple and papaya (in moderation). Pineapple contains the digestive enzyme bromelain, while papaya is rich in papain.

MSM is one of the most powerful anti-inflammatories derived from natural foods. This non-toxic, active sulfur compound may facilitate the production of certain enzymes needed to counteract inflammation. I suggest taking ½ teaspoon of MSM granules once or twice a day, with meals.

Quercetin, a bioflavonoid found most abundantly in apples and onions, has been found to be highly effective in lowering inflammation by inhibiting the release of histamines and other inflammatory substances such

Rev Up Your Metabolism

Ever wonder why slim people stay slim and fat people stay fat? A key factor is what I call "energy conversion." Food broken down in the digestive tract is absorbed into the bloodstream and dispersed into cells throughout the body where it fuels energy. In lean people, heat production goes up by as much as 40 percent after a meal, which means they're burning the fuel. In overweight people, it may rise 10 percent or less, which means food energy is stored as fat rather than burned.

Convert Fat to Energy

There are natural nutritional supplements you can take to activate your nervous system and increase your metabolic rate to encourage dietary fat's conversion to energy, rather than storage as body fat. Following are some of the most powerful metabolism-boosters.

Green tea contains polyphenols, which in addition to having powerful antioxidant and cancer-prevention properties, wake up your body's ability to burn calories. I recommend drinking at least three eight-ounce cups daily (to provide roughly 240–320 mg of polyphenols). If you prefer not to drink the tea, try 300–400 mg daily of green tea extract (be sure the product is caffeine-free and standardized to 80 percent total polyphenol and 55 percent epigallocatechin), or 100 mg of green tea polyphenols, taken three times daily.

L-Carnitine occurs naturally in your body. Its job is to bind to fatty acids and transport them into your mitochondria—your cells' fuel-burning furnaces—where

as leukotrienes, which are one thousand times more potent in stimulating inflammation than histamines are. I recommend taking 300–600 mg of quercetin once or twice a day. To increase absorption rate, be sure to take with 500–1,000 mg of bromelain.

Finally, vitamin C reduces inflammation by decreasing histamine levels in the blood, and aiding in the production of adrenal corticosteroids—your body's own anti-inflammatory agents. For inflammatory conditions, I recommend taking 3,000–5,000 mg of buffered vitamin C each day. Buffered vitamin C, as well as the other recommended nutritional supplements, has minimal to no side effects and is available in most natural food or health food stores.

the fatty acids are burned to produce adenosine triphosphate (ATP), your body's primary source of energy. One side effect of L-carnitine deficiency is that food is stored as fat instead of being used as energy. This not only lowers your energy levels, but it also makes it difficult for you to lose weight.

Recent studies have shown that people who eat a well-balanced diet, exercise moderately, and supplement with L-carnitine every day lose an average of 25 percent more weight than people who do not take L-carnitine. This makes sense, because through supplementation, your mitochondria get the fuel they need to produce energy, allowing your body to burn more calories (from fat) at the same time.

Many women are carnitine-deficient, especially vegetarians and those in mid-life and beyond. Red meat is the best source of carnitine, but too much red meat can disrupt the acid/alkaline balance that is so important to overall good health. I recommend 1,000 mg of L-carnitine per day in divided doses, half in the morning and half at night. Side effects are rare and occur mostly with a dosage of more than 1,000 mg at a time. There are no known contraindications with pharmaceutical drugs or other nutritional supplements. If you do experience gastric upset or diarrhea, cut your dosage by half for better tolerance.

L-Tyrosine: One in four American women can attribute their weight gain to low or borderline-low thyroid hormones. When the thyroid gland is functioning properly, it produces hormones that regulate metabolism and convert food into energy. Women with poor thyroid function or hypothyroidism don't burn calories efficiently and experience fatigue, weakness, depression, weight gain, and high cholesterol

levels. Many doctors ignore the nutritional supplements that can help correct thyroid dysfunction, such as the amino acid L-tyrosine, which is used by your body to produce thyroid hormones and also helps rev up your metabolism, allowing you to burn more calories each day.

L-tyrosine is so vital to all energy interactions that I often include it in my nutritional programs for women with chronic fatigue, whether due to stress, poor nutrition, or the aging process. And because L-tyrosine is converted into excitatory neurotransmitters—chemicals within your brain that boost physical stamina, mental acuity, and enthusiasm for life—it's just the kind of lift you need while dieting.

Balance Blood Sugar

Every time you gain weight, your "set point" is nudged up. That's the point at which the calories you consume equal the calories you expend, and it's related to insulin sensitivity. Insulin enables blood sugar, or glucose, to move from your bloodstream into your cells, to be used for energy. Blood sugar cannot enter cells when they become insensitive or resistant to insulin. The result: Declining energy, declining ability to burn fat, as well as more pounds due to increasing storage of new fat, converted from the excess glucose.

The biggest cause of insulin resistance is a diet high in refined sugar and simple carbohydrates, such as sugar, white breads, white rice, pasta made from refined flour, cakes, and cookies. Strengthening your body's ability to use insulin helps reestablish normal metabolism, and helps you turn glucose into energy more efficiently.

One way to help restore healthy glucose metabolism is to correct your body's chromium deficiency. Chromium is essential for protein, carbohydrate, and fat metabolism. And, it increases the number of binding sites for insulin on cells, providing more ways for glucose to enter cells to be transformed into energy. Unfortunately, the typical American diet is high in refined foods and simple sugars and low in chromium. In one study, dieting women given chromium polynicotinate experienced greater fat loss and maintained lean body mass better than women who didn't receive chromium. Research also suggests chromium's effects may be long term, providing benefits even after you stop taking it. I recommend 200–400 mcg of chromium picolinate per day.

Rebalance Your Life

Of course, body chemistry is only half of the picture. Your lifestyle is a factor too. Your activity level, stress level, and food choices play a large role in determining whether you're able to attain and maintain your optimal weight, by influencing whether what you eat is stored in your body or burned as fuel. It's time to focus on what you eat, how you burn it, and how you deal with stress.

Exercise for Weight Loss

Regular aerobic exercise, combined with strength training, gives you a natural metabolic boost. As such, exercise is one of the key tools you can use to achieve and maintain your optimal weight. First of all, aerobic exercise directly burns calories. And, the more muscle you have from strength training, the more calories you burn, not only while doing aerobic exercise but even when you're doing nothing more strenuous than sitting at the kitchen table reading the paper. That's because it takes energy to keep those lovely, lean muscles alive. It's called the "thermogenic effect."

The benefits of both kinds of exercise are numerous, including burning more calories, reducing cravings, and improving your overall emotional well being. Exercise even helps you think more clearly and move with more physical grace, thanks to improved oxygenation and circulation to your brain and nerves, which not only provides more nutrients to those vital tissues but also clears out more toxins and debris.

Additionally, exercise increases production of neurochemicals like dopamine and beta-endorphins. These natural substances greatly improve alertness and produce a sense of elation and well-being, while reducing anxiety and depression and enabling you to cope better with stress.

Exercise also improves the function of your thyroid gland, protecting your body against thyroid hormone imbalances as you age.

Here are few ideas for exercise that are enjoyable, good for you, and don't require a lot of time or money.

Aerobic Exercise

My all time favorite aerobic exercise is walking. It not only improves your cardiovascular health and helps you lose weight, but because it requires a larger array of your body's muscles to walk than it does to run, it works its healthful magic as efficiently as more strenuous exercise does, and without the heightened risks of injury and wear-and-tear. Researchers at the Washington University School of Medicine in St. Louis put a group of men and women, aged 60–70, on a 9- to 12-month exercise program that consisted of either walking or jogging. On average, the subjects exercised 45 minutes three to five times per week. By the end of the study, they'd all lost weight, mostly in their abdominal area.

If you haven't been exercising regularly, don't jump into it all at once. Remember, it takes three weeks to make a habit, and we want long-term results. The best path to that goal is to establish the exercise habit first. Start slowly, with a 15-minute walk, then gradually build up until you're walking 30–45 minutes three to five times a week. If you're already at this level, try adding hills or stairs to your routine.

Strength-Training (Non-Aerobic) Exercise

I also like non-aerobic exercises, like Pilates. It's similar to yoga in that you do a series of exercises designed to stretch and strengthen your muscles and joints. But while yoga is based on the flow of energy through your body, Pilates focuses on physical conditioning and body toning.

If you're well-muscled and well-hydrated, with strong and healthy joints, try Power Yoga. This is a combination of deep breathing with specifically sequenced sets of flowing yoga postures. It helps you build strength, increase endurance, release tension, and create more flexibility in your entire body while also providing more of an aerobic workout than other forms of yoga. However, Power Yoga can be dehydrating. Therefore, if you tend towards excess bloat and fluid retention, I suggest you try other forms of yoga. Your best bet for yoga is to find a class at your local YMCA or gym. Try to take the class two or three times a week.

Finding the Time

While many of the women that I've worked with over the years do participate in regular exercise, some do not, claiming that they'd like to, but simply don't have the time. I have two responses to that. First, you don't need a huge chunk of time to exercise. It takes 3,500 calories to equal a pound of weight. So if you want to lose a pound, you need a combination of nutritional changes and exercise that will allow you to either burn 3,500 calories, or take in 3,500 fewer calories, each week—or 500 calories a day. That's not as difficult as it might sound. Simply cutting out one regular soft drink a day, and taking a 45-minute brisk walk, is all it'll take. Second, it's not about time, it's about how important your health is to you.

The Stress Connection

Let's say you had a tense one-on-one with your boss, your teenager brought home a "D" in calculus, and your husband is heading out the door on another business trip, leaving you with a flooded basement and three soccer games in two days. If you're like many women, your way of handling the stress is to hit the freezer for a pint of Cherry Garcia, raid the kids' holiday candy, or order in an extra large meat lovers' pizza—and then devour the entire thing in one sitting. Often called "unconscious eating," this kind of stress-related eating is a major contributor to many women's weight gain.

However, stress affects your weight—and your health—in more insidious ways than overeating. Whenever you're feeling stressed—whether it's while stuck in traffic or while going through a divorce—your body reacts as if it were preparing to fight an angry tiger. Chemical signals from your brain increase your breathing rate in an effort to bring in more oxygen, divert blood away from your digestive system to your muscles and brain, and trigger a release of energy-enhancing glucose, while mobilizing carbohydrates and stored fat for quick energy. It all happens automatically, and you may be so accustomed to it that you're not even aware it's happening.

Ideally, this chemical response should give you the energy and voom to escape that tiger. And, ideally, this type of chemical response should only be necessary once in a while. After all, there aren't tigers looming around every corner! The problem is that in our world today, the tigers are everywhere, in the form of traffic jams, deadlines, demands, conflicts, and bills—highly significant stresses, but not the kind that require a physical battle or a 10-mile sprint, which would burn off a lot of the glucose that flooded your bloodstream on cue from those chemical stress signals. Instead, the glucose remains in your bloodstream, triggering the release of insulin, which in turn converts that extra glucose into fat, generally packing it on around your abdomen, where the fat cells have greater than the average number of receptors for stress hormones.

That's why it's so important that you add stress-reduction techniques to your life if you want to lose weight and be healthier in general. Exercise is one fabulous technique, because it releases stress-busting hormones like endorphins. Here are some other techniques I use and recommend for everyone.

Deep Breathing

I'm sure you think you know how to breathe. But you may not know how to breathe to reduce stress. This takes deep abdominal breathing—a more effective way to carry oxygen, the fuel for metabolic activity, to all tissues of your body. Shallow breathing, which is what you do when you're engaged in chronically stressful activities, can leave your tissues under-oxygenated. This makes you fatigued and unable to burn calories efficiently. Deep breathing helps relax your entire body and strengthens the muscles in your chest and abdomen. Do this deep breathing exercise for three to five minutes every hour and whenever you're feeling tense:

1. Lie flat on your back with your knees pulled up. Keep your feet slightly apart. (If you're in a situation where you can't get the privacy to assume this position, simply adjust your sitting position, uncross your legs, place your feet squarely on the floor, and continue the exercise.)
2. Inhale deeply through your nose. As you breathe in, allow your stomach to relax so the air flows into your abdomen. Your stomach should balloon out as you breathe in.
3. Visualize your lungs filling up with energy so your chest swells out.
4. Exhale deeply. As you breathe out, let your stomach and chest collapse. Imagine the air coming out from your abdomen and then from your lungs.

Visualization

With visualization, you create a soothing and relaxing picture in your mind. Try to make the image as detailed as possible. If you're on a beach, feel the sand between your toes, smell the seawater, and luxuriate in the caress of the breeze on your sun-kissed skin.

Laughter

Laughter has been shown—scientifically—to lower circulating levels of the stress hormone cortisol as well as the blood pressure and heart rate, and to increase mood-elevating beta-endorphins. So spend a night watching old sit-coms, the Comedy Channel, or rent a couple of comedies. The point is, make a point of laughing. Pop some air-popcorn (sans butter!) and prepare to giggle.

Spirituality and Prayer

Countless people over the centuries have turned to prayer for a sense of safety and calm; and a growing body of evidence points to the beneficial health effects of prayer and spirituality. This doesn't mean you have to be religious. You can find spirituality during a walk in the woods on a fall day, listening to an inspiring piece of music, or simply sitting before a lighted candle and doing some deep breathing and meditation exercises. Make spiritual practice a new habit, for physical and emotional health and stress reduction.

Aromatherapy

The essential oils of plants can help counteract stress, an aspect of herbal medicine called aromatherapy. Essential oils may enter the body by inhaling them, using vaporizers, steam inhalations, diffusers, or even a tissue dampened with a drop of oil held to the nose. They can also be absorbed through massage and/or soaking in warm bath water infused with a few drops of an essential oil. Those particularly beneficial for

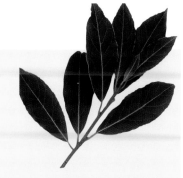

**Sniff Away
Your Appetite**

The powers of scents and smell amaze me. For years, I have used aromatherapy to help me relax and to alleviate certain symptoms. But research also indicates that it can help you eat less by making you feel fuller and more satisfied after your meal.

An easy and inexpensive way to use aromatherapy to control your appetite is to simply purchase apple- (preferably green apple), banana-, or peppermint-scented flavorings from a health food store or the spice department of specialty supermarkets. Just sniff them three times in each nostril whenever you want to curb your appetite.

Other helpful tips to help control your appetite include:

→   Smell your food before you eat it.
→   Limit your food choices at any one meal. In other words, forego the buffet.
→   Opt for fresh food rather than pre-packaged or canned food.
→   Eat hot or warm food rather than cold, since foods' natural aromas are more efficiently released when food is warm.
→   Choose the most aromatic foods, such as those containing garlic, onions, herbs, and spices.

stress include lavender, chamomile, orange, tangerine, lemon, rose, spruce, and ylang ylang. Try using a diffuser in your office, putting a drop of lavender oil on your pillow at night, or soaking in an aromatic bath when you feel tense.

Top 5 Foods for Boosting Metabolism

There are many wonderful foods that are not only healthy and delicious, but will also kick your metabolism into high gear. Here are five of them:

Green Tea

Green tea contains special chemicals called polyphenols, which have exceptional antioxidant activity and help promote overall good health and well-being. One cup of brewed green tea contains about 100 mg of polyphenols. While there isn't enough research to call green tea a "diet miracle," one research study suggests that green tea is effective in helping to burn calories. Specifically, researchers divided participants into three groups, giving them either a placebo, caffeine, or green tea extract. They found that those who received the green tea burned an additional 500 calories per week, with no changes in diet or physical activity. They also burned more fat than either the placebo or caffeine groups.

Why does it work? The polyphenols in green tea appear to block the enzyme that breaks down norepinephrine, a brain chemical related to metabolism. The higher your levels of norepinephrine, the greater your metabolism and the faster you'll burn calories.

Almonds

The oil in almonds contains phenylethylamine, a naturally occurring, feel-good brain chemical that works as a natural metabolism booster. Phenylethylamine works similarly to amphetamines by revving up your metabolism (without any of the anxiety, shakiness, and other negative side effects of the drug). Phenylethylamine is also thought to play a role in improving your mood and energy, both of which are important in controlling your eating, by providing the motivation you need to become more physically active.

Garbanzo Beans (Chickpeas)

Garbanzo beans contain L-phenylalanine, an essential amino acid that functions as a natural antidepressant and improves memory, mood, and libido, as well as boosting your metabolism. L-phenylalanine helps get you moving in the morning, clears your mind, and improves your mental clarity, allowing you to focus on things other than losing weight. Additionally, L-phenylalanine provides a feeling of fullness, enabling you to eat less and still feel satisfied.

Other foods that contain L-phenylalanine include soybeans, fish, poultry, almonds, pecans, pumpkin and sesame seeds, lima beans, and lentils.

Tofu

By increasing your consumption of tofu, you'll actually increase your levels of L-tyrosine, as soy is extremely high in this amino acid. In addition to boosting physical stamina, mental energy, and sharpness, tyrosine helps your body produce thyroid hormones that drive your metabolism and help to burn calories and regulate your weight much more efficiently.

By helping to maintain healthy thyroid function, tyrosine works to keep your weight and hunger under control. As an added bonus, it improves your sex drive and has been shown to promote an overall sense of well-being. Other foods that contain L-tyrosine include fish and poultry.

Brown Rice

Lastly, I would encourage you to include lots of brown rice in your diet. Whole grains such as brown rice are high in chromium, a mineral that is essential for metabolizing protein, carbohydrates, and fats. It also increases your body's own natural sensitivity to insulin, thus aiding in your weight loss efforts.

In fact, animal studies have shown that chromium deficiency negatively affects glucose intolerance, fat metabolism, protein synthesis, and longevity. It has also been shown to help increase lean body mass and decrease the percentage of body fat—both factors in weight loss.

Weight Loss Recipes

You've got to eat to lose weight. Strange but true. The trick is to eat the right foods, in the right amounts. So, dig in to the following recipes, starring high-fiber, nutrient-rich foods with metabolism-boosting ingredients. Based on my pH-balance philosophy, they'll truly help you in your quest for weight loss and health maintenance, plus they're truly satisfying and delicious.

Shakes & Drinks

Chilly Dilly Cucumber Concoction Serves 1

Cucumbers provide only 13 calories per 4 ounces. Their flesh contains vitamin C, while their fiber-rich skin boasts a variety of minerals, including silica, potassium, and magnesium.

    1 piece frozen cucumber (about 3 ounces), remove peel and seeds
    3 small sprigs fresh dill
    1 teaspoon lemon juice
    ¼ cup soy yogurt
    ½ cup cold non-dairy kefir (e.g., SoyTreat)
    2 tablespoons rice protein powder
    Salt to taste
    Black pepper to taste
    1 slice cucumber

Dice the frozen cucumber and put it in a blender.

Wash and shake dry the dill and set aside 1 sprig for garnish. Remove the leaves from the stems of the remaining two sprigs, chop the leaves coarsely, and put them in the blender with the lemon juice, yogurt, and half of the non-dairy kefir. Blend well for 15 seconds. Add the rice protein powder and the remaining ¼ cup of kefir. Season with salt and pepper, and blend for another 10 seconds.

Pour the concoction over ice in a glass. Partially slit the cucumber slice and fit it onto the glass rim with the reserved dill. Serve with a straw.

Mango Lassi Serves 2

The mango in this traditional South Asian yogurt drink is loaded with folic acid, which supports your adrenal glands to enhance energy and stamina, supports normal cholesterol levels, and supports the health of your brain and nervous system.

2 ½ cups plain, dairy-free yogurt
1 teaspoon lemon juice
1 cup fresh mango pulp
⅔ cup cold water
8 tablespoons honey
18–20 standard-sized ice cubes

Blend the first five ingredients in the blender until the honey is dissolved. Add the ice and blend until frothy.

Naked Papaya Breeze Serves 2

Tropical fruits—such as papaya, pineapple, and mango—brim with enzymes that chauffeur fat burners to your cells' doorsteps.

¾ cup cubed, peeled papaya
¾ cup cubed fresh pineapple
½ medium carrot, peeled
1 cup chilled papaya juice
½ tablespoon minced, peeled fresh ginger
½ tablespoon fresh lime juice
½ tablespoon honey

Skin and cube the papaya and pineapple and peel and grate the carrot. Place all ingredients in a blender; process until smooth.

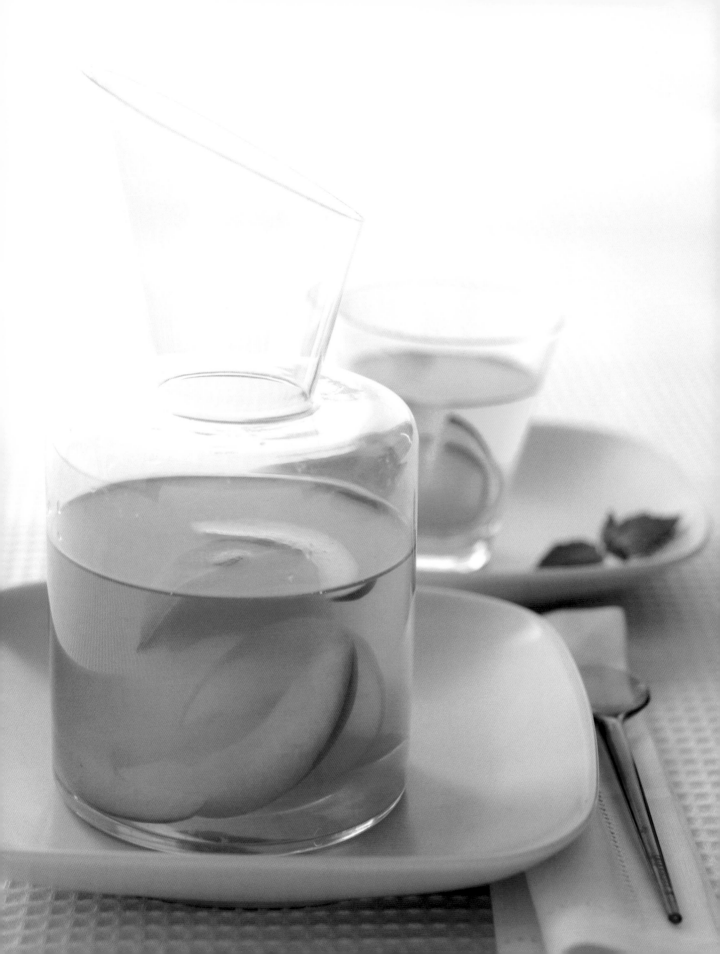

Iced Peachy Green Tea Serves 2

This simple and delicious brew, featuring green tea's metabolism-boosting polyphenols, is just the thing to cool you off and slim you down—all at once!

1 ripe peach
2 cups water
2 green tea bags
Xylitol to taste
Mint sprigs

Wash, pit, and slice the peach, and put it in a saucepan with the water. Bring to a brisk boil, then pour water and peaches over teabags.

Let steep for 6 minutes. Allow tea to cool, then refrigerate until thoroughly cool.

Pour tea, including peach slices, into two glasses. Add xylitol to taste. Serve each glass with a spoon and a sprig of fresh mint.

Pineapple Strawberry Cooler   Serves 1

This liquid treat blends two high-fiber sources: strawberries, with their cholesterol-leveling pectin and fat-burning vitamin C, and pineapple, with its protein-digesting enzyme, bromelain.

    3 ounces strawberries
    2 teaspoons lemon juice
    1 teaspoon floral honey
    ⅔ cup cold pineapple juice
    2 tablespoons rice protein powder

Gently wash and hull all strawberries, setting aside one strawberry for garnish. Quarter the hulled berries and put them, with the lemon juice, honey, and half the pineapple juice into a blender and whiz thoroughly for 15 seconds.

Add the rice protein powder and the remaining pineapple juice and blend for another 10 seconds.

Pour the concoction into a tall glass. Partially slit the reserved strawberry and fit it onto the glass rim for garnish. Serve with a straw.

Strawberry & Kiwi Minty Milkshake   Serves 2

Phenol-rich strawberries are a heart-protective fruit, an anti-cancer fruit, and an anti-inflammatory fruit, all in one red, heart-shaped berry.

1 kiwi
3–4 ounces fresh strawberries
2 teaspoons chopped fresh mint
1 tablespoon fresh lime juice
2 teaspoons maple syrup
2 tablespoons quick-cooking oatmeal
½ cup soy yogurt
½ cup cold rice or nut milk

Halve the kiwi and squeeze the flesh from the peel into a blender. Gently rinse and hull the strawberries. Put the strawberries, mint, lime juice, maple syrup, oatmeal, and soy yogurt into the blender and purée for about 15 seconds. Pour in the milk and purée until smooth, adding a little more milk if necessary for consistency.

Pour into two large glasses and sip shakes with wide straws.

Sweet Dreams Tea   Serves 2

Since kava helps to relax your muscles and valerian root calms your mood, you'll find this tea hits the spot after a long, stressful day.

1 pint water
1 teaspoon dried kava leaves
1 teaspoon dried valerian root leaves
1 teaspoon xylitol (optional)

Bring the water to a boil. Place herbs in water and stir. Reduce heat to low and steep for 15 minutes. Add xylitol, if desired.

Spicy Veggie Cocktail   Serves 2

This drink is great when it comes to burning fat, but that's not all. Did you know that celery root, AKA celeriac, has diuretic properties, stimulates the appetite, aids digestion, and supports the lymphatic, nervous, and urinary systems?

    3 ounces red bell pepper
    3 ounces celery root (celeriac)
    2 tablespoons chopped fresh Italian parsley
    ½ teaspoon crushed red pepper flakes
    1 ¼ cups cold V8 juice
    Salt to taste
    Black pepper to taste

Wash and core the bell pepper and remove its seeds. Scrub and peel the celery root. Dice root and bell pepper, and put both, with parsley, red pepper flakes, and ½ cup V8 juice, in a blender and purée.

Add the remaining V8 juice and purée until smooth. Season with salt and pepper.

Pour the cocktail over ice cubes in two glasses, and serve with wide straws.

Snacks & Appetizers

Almonds

For a very quick and simple snack on the go, grab a handful of almonds. Almond oil contains phenylethylamine, which works similarly to amphetamines by revving your metabolism (without the anxiety, shakes, or other negative side effects of the drug). The substance also plays a role in revving your mood and energy, providing the motivation you need to become more physically active.

Fight sweet cravings with a handful of raw or unsalted almonds. Snacks that contain healthy oils and protein and complex carbohydrates cause blood sugar to rise, peak, and drop slowly, thereby controlling cravings.

Arugula Pâté   Serves 2

A member of the Brassica family with cabbage and broccoli, arugula is a rich source of iron and vitamins A and C, and contains plant compounds that lower a woman's risk of breast cancer.

   3 ounces arugula
   2 tablespoons pumpkin seeds
   2 tablespoons freshly grated soy Parmesan cheese
   2 teaspoons balsamic vinegar
   2 tablespoons olive oil
   4–5 tablespoons vegetable stock
   Salt to taste
   Black pepper to taste
   1 green onion
   2 pieces rye crisp bread

Rinse, shake dry, and chop the arugula; then place it, the pumpkin seeds, Parmesan, vinegar, and olive oil in a food processor and purée until smooth. Stir in the stock to form a creamy paste, and season with salt and pepper. Finely slice the green onion into rings, and gently fold it into the paste.

Spread on rye crisps.

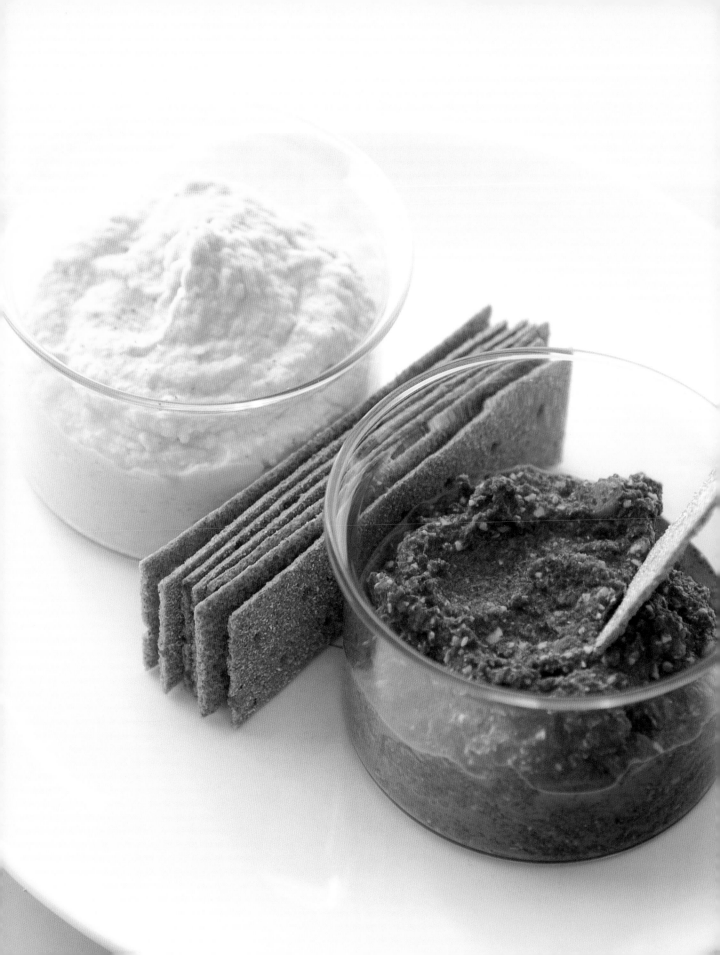

Hummus   Makes about 5 ½ cups

Garbanzo beans are excellent sources of low-fat protein, fiber, and complex carbohydrates. Hummus is also rich in the B vitamins essential for regulation of hormone levels and critical to just about every body function.

4 cups garbanzo beans
½ cup tahini (sesame seed paste)
⅓ cup warm water
⅓ cup olive oil
Juice of 1 lemon
4–5 garlic cloves
1 ½ teaspoons salt
2 teaspoons cumin
Pepper to taste

Combine garbanzo beans, tahini, water, olive oil, and lemon in a blender or food processor and process until smooth and creamy. Add garlic, salt, cumin, and pepper.

Process again and serve.

See page 100 for recipe of Arugula Pâté also shown on opposite page.

Savory Zucchini Sauté Serves 2

More than 95 percent water, zucchini is a great, low calorie vegetable. Its fiber helps fill you up and keep you feeling full, while its wide variety of female-beneficial nutrients, including potassium and phosphorus, help keep your body in a slightly alkaline state.

3 ounces white mushrooms
1 green onion
2 teaspoons fresh lemon juice
1 teaspoon balsamic vinegar
1 ½ tablespoons olive oil
2 teaspoons toasted sesame seeds
Salt to taste
Black pepper to taste
8 ounces large zucchini

Rinse and stem the mushrooms, then slice them and the green onion. Toss them in the lemon juice, vinegar, 1 tablespoon of the olive oil, sesame seeds, salt, and pepper. Rinse the zucchini, slice into eight medallions, and season with salt.

Brush the remaining olive oil in a skillet and heat to medium. Sauté the zucchini medallions for a few minutes on each side, and season with salt and pepper.

Transfer the zucchini to plates and top with the mushroom mixture.

Cumin-Get-It Popcorn Serves 8

Popcorn is loaded with fiber and has only 108 calories per 2 quarts of air-popped corn.

1 tablespoon olive oil
1 teaspoon Bragg Liquid Aminos
16 cups air-popped popcorn (from ¾ cup popcorn kernels)
1 ½ teaspoons ground cumin
1 teaspoon ground coriander

Mix olive oil and Bragg Liquid Aminos and add slowly to popcorn, drizzling over the kernels. Add remaining ingredients and toss well.

Tropical Fruit Salsa   Makes 2 cups

This vitamin-packed salsa also features papaya's digestive enzyme, papain, and pineapple's bromelain, which act as natural anti-inflammatories.

½ cup diced mango
½ cup diced peeled papaya
½ cup diced fresh pineapple
½ cup diced Granny Smith apple
¼ cup diced red bell pepper
¼ cup thinly sliced green onions
1 tablespoon minced fresh cilantro
1 tablespoon xylitol
1 tablespoon orange juice
¼ teaspoon crushed red pepper
⅛ teaspoon ground cumin

Peel the mango and papaya and dice them along with the pineapple, apple, and bell pepper. Rinse and thinly slice on the diagonal the green onions. Rinse and shake dry the cilantro and mince.

Combine all ingredients in a bowl. Mix well. Let stand at room temperature at least 1 hour.

Serve this salsa with tortilla chips or as a fabulous accompaniment to just about anything, but particularly with grilled or sautéed fish.

Turkey & Herb Dip with Crudités Serves 2

By increasing consumption of tofu, you'll increase your levels of L-tyrosine, an amino acid, which helps your body produce thyroid hormones that drive metabolism, help burn calories, and regulate weight more efficiently. Plus, it perks up your sex drive!

2 ounces turkey
Handful of fresh herbs (e.g., basil, oregano, and/or thyme)
¼ lemon
3 tablespoons chopped almonds
½ cup silken tofu
Salt to taste
Black pepper to taste
1 head Belgian endive
½ small bunch celery
1 small zucchini
1 carrot
1 small kohlrabi
1 small red bell pepper

Dice the turkey. Wash and shake dry the herbs, plucking leaves away from stalks. Reserve a few leaves for garnish and chop the rest. Rinse the lemon in hot water and dry. Grate the zest and squeeze the juice, including pulp.

Mix the turkey, herbs, lemon zest, lemon juice to taste, almonds, and silken tofu. Blend well and season with salt and pepper to taste.

Remove the endive's outer leaves, halve and core it, then separate into individual leaves. Wash and trim the remaining vegetables. Cut them into dippable sticks.

Arrange all vegetables on a platter, with the dip in the center. Garnish with the reserved herbs and serve.

Turkey-Wrapped & Basil-Dipped Asparagus   Serves 2

Basil's flavonoids and volatile oils have anti-bacterial properties and produce anti-inflammatory effects. The vitamin A-rich green leaves possess nutrients essential for cardiovascular health, as well.

10 ounces asparagus
1 teaspoon olive oil
½ cup soy yogurt
2 tablespoons dairy-free sour cream
1 teaspoon capers, drained
1 teaspoon fresh lemon juice
Salt to taste
Black pepper to taste
12 leaves fresh basil
2 ounces smoked turkey, sliced

Rinse the asparagus, snap off the tough ends, and peel the bottom third of the spears. In a saucepan, bring to boil a large quantity of water and the oil. Add the asparagus spears, cover, reduce heat, and simmer until crisp-tender, about 10–12 minutes.

To prepare the dip, mix the soy yogurt and sour cream. Mince the capers and stir them in. Season the dip with lemon juice, salt, and pepper.

Wash and shake dry the basil and reserve several leaves for garnish. Finely chop the remaining leaves and stir them into the dip.

Drain the asparagus, give it a cold-water bath to stop the cooking, and drain again.

Wrap the turkey around the asparagus spears and arrange on a platter. Serve with the dip, garnishing with the reserved basil.

Breakfast

Broccoli Frittata   Serves 2

This Italian egg white omelet makes a great brunch dish. And since it's cooked in olive oil, you gain a great source of essential fatty acids, which substantially lower your risk of heart disease by lowering LDL cholesterol and triglycerides.

　　1 cup chopped onions (about 1 medium onion)
　　2 cups chopped broccoli (about ½-inch pieces)
　　2 teaspoons chopped fresh basil (1 teaspoon dried)
　　1 tablespoon olive oil
　　2 garlic cloves, minced or pressed
　　Salt and black pepper to taste
　　6 egg whites
　　¼ cup grated dairy-free pecorino or mozzarella

Preheat broiler.

Peel and chop the onion. Rinse, shake dry, and chop the broccoli and basil. In a large, ovenproof skillet, heat the olive oil and sauté the onions for 5 minutes, until tender. Add the broccoli, garlic, and basil and sauté for another 5 minutes, stirring occasionally, until the broccoli is crisp-tender but still vivid green.

Combine the salt, pepper, and egg whites and whisk until frothy. Pour the froth over the broccoli, tilting the skillet so the egg whites flow evenly throughout the broccoli. Cook on low for 3–4 minutes, until egg whites are opaque and close to firm.

Sprinkle grated dairy-free cheese over egg mixture, and place skillet under the broiler for 2–3 minutes, until cheese has melted and begins to brown. Halve the frittata and serve.

Mixed Berry Pistachio Parfait   Serves 2

Nuts, such as pistachios, are great sources of healthful polyunsaturated fats; the B-complex vitamins; vitamins A, D, and E; and a wealth of minerals, including calcium, potassium, magnesium, iron, copper, zinc, and phosphorous.

    9 ounces mixed berries or red grapes
    2 teaspoons lemon juice
    1 tablespoon unfiltered, organic apple juice
    4 teaspoons chopped pistachios
    1 ¼ cups soy or rice yogurt

Gently rinse and drain the fruit. Cut larger berries and/or grapes into bite-sized pieces. Toss with lemon and apple juices. Finely chop the pistachios and combine them with the yogurt.

In small glasses or parfait dishes, alternate layers of fruit and yogurt, ending with a final layer of fruit.

No-Cook Red Currant-Strawberry Jam   Makes 1 jar (10 ounces)

This honey-sweetened, alkaline-forming, uncooked jam retains all the raw fruits' vitamins. Red currants are an outstanding source of beta carotene, B vitamins, and vitamin C, as well as potassium and calcium.

    8 ounces red currants
    4 ounces strawberries
    ⅓–½ cup honey

Gently rinse and drain the currants and strawberries. Remove the currants from their stems and press them through a coarse sieve. Cut large strawberries into smaller pieces. With an electric mixer, beat the currant purée, strawberries, and honey to taste for 10 minutes, until the mixture starts to thicken.

Store in a tightly capped, sterilized jar in a cool, dark place for 4–6 weeks. Refrigerate when opened and consume as soon as possible.

Serve mixed into soy yogurt, or atop whole-grain, wheat-free waffles or toast. Lovely with Potato-Spelt Bread (see recipe on page 111).

Smoked Salmon on Mock Rye with Apple-Horseradish Spread   Serves 2

Apples are high in quercetin, a bioflavonoid effective in lowering inflammation and inhibiting the release of histamines and other inflammatory substances.

2 tablespoons dairy-free cream cheese (e.g., Soya Kaas or Tofutti)
1 teaspoon grated fresh horseradish
Black pepper to taste
⅓ medium apple (e.g., Northern Spy, Gala, Winesap, or Granny Smith)
2 teaspoons lemon juice
2 slices gluten-free rye bread (such as Enjoy Life Foods Rye-less Rye Bread)
2 sprigs fresh dill
2 ounces smoked salmon

Stir the cream cheese with the horseradish and a pinch of pepper. Cut the apple into thin slices and sprinkle it with the lemon juice.

Spread the horseradish blend onto the bread slices and halve them diagonally. Wash and shake dry the dill.

Arrange even portions of the apple slices, salmon, and dill on the bread. Enjoy.

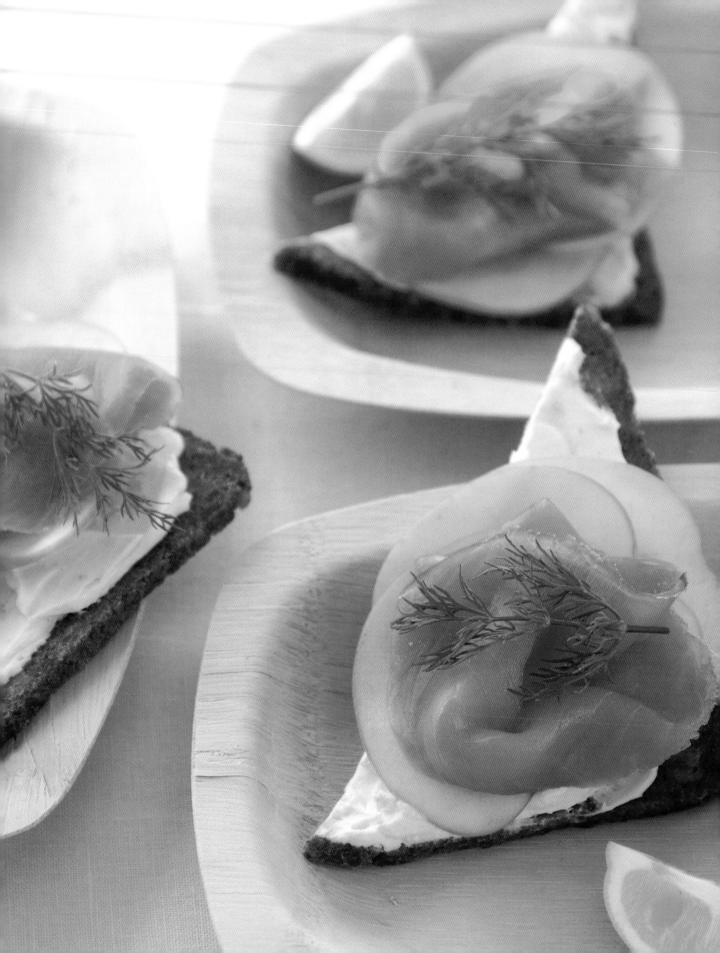

Poached Huevos Rancheros   Serves 2

This poached take on huevos rancheros features flaxseed oil, which is rich in alpha linolenic acid, an omega-3 fatty acid. Omega-3s prevent obesity and improve insulin response, among other health benefits.

2 eggs
Olive oil spray
2 tablespoons chopped cilantro
2 teaspoons flaxseed oil
2 corn tortillas
⅔ cup cooked brown rice
½ cup cooked pinto beans
2 tablespoons grated non-dairy cheese (e.g., rice or soy cheese)

Add water to a large skillet, filling two-thirds full. Bring to a boil; reduce heat, and simmer. Break eggs into 2 (6-ounce each) custard cups coated with olive oil spray. Place custard cups in simmering water in skillet. Cover skillet; cook 6 minutes.

While eggs are poaching, rinse, shake dry, and chop the cilantro. Remove custard cups from water.

Heat 1 teaspoon of flaxseed oil in large skillet over medium heat. Place tortilla in skillet and place a thin layer of rice, and then beans on top of tortilla. Add 1 poached egg and half of the grated cheese. Reduce flame to low. Cook for 1 more minute. Repeat process to create second huevo ranchero and serve.

Potato-Spelt Bread Makes 2 loaves

An ancient cereal grain that is easily digestible, spelt is an excellent source of vitamin B2, a very good source of manganese, and a good source of niacin, thiamin, and copper.

1 pound baking potatoes
2 pounds whole-grain spelt flour
2 packets rapid-rise yeast
Lukewarm water
2 tablespoons salt
1 teaspoon ground cumin
2 ounces toasted sesame seeds
8 ounces sunflower seeds

Steam the potatoes 20–30 minutes, until tender. Peel while still hot and push through a potato ricer into a large bowl. Sift together the spelt flours and the yeast, and add them gradually to the mashed potatoes, mixing well. If the dough is too stiff, thin it with a little water. It should be soft and pliant. Shape it into a ball in the bowl. Cover and let the dough rise at room temperature for 1 hour.

Knead in gently the salt, cumin, and half of each of the seeds. Grease two loaf pans and sprinkle with half of the remaining seeds. Place the loaves in the bottom of a cold oven, heat to 400°F, and bake about 1 hour, when the firm loaves have shrunken from the sides of the pans and have a hollow sound when thumped on the bottom. Cool the bread in the pans, then remove.

Serve with No-Cook Red Currant-Strawberry Jam (see recipe page 107).

Baking Soda is Not for Cookies Alone

Baking soda, also known as sodium bicarbonate, is an effective buffering agent that helps neutralize the overacidity of most holiday meals by relieving acid indigestion, sour stomach, and heartburn. Take ¼–½ teaspoon in 4-ounces of water an hour and a half after eating. If you are concerned about excessive sodium intake, on a sodium-restricted diet, are pregnant, or are taking heart medications, speak with your physician before taking large amounts of sodium bicarbonate.

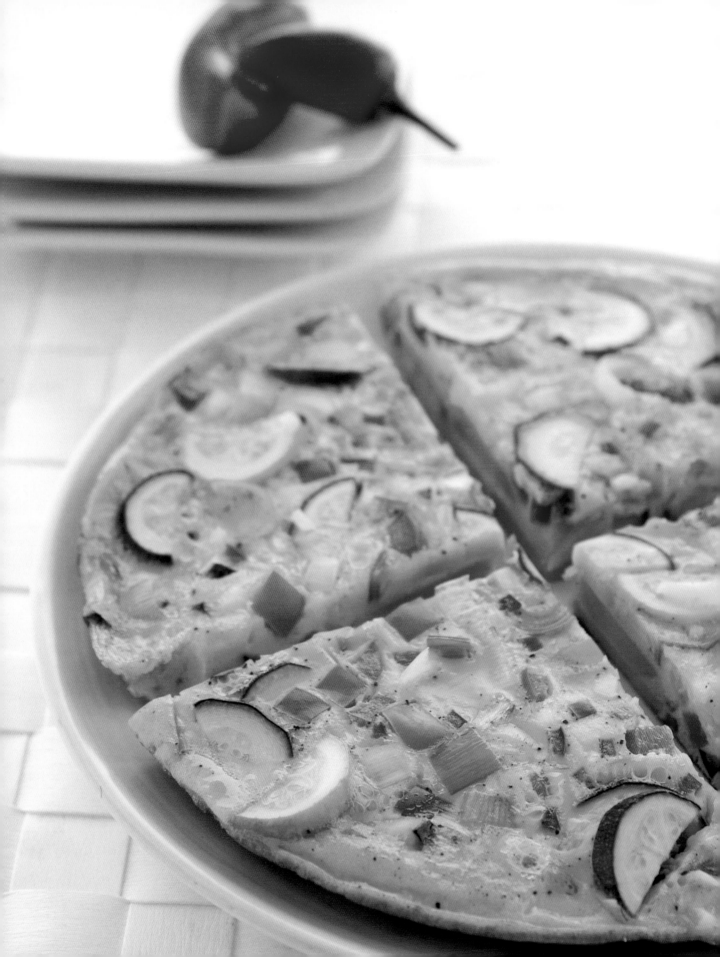

Tortilla Española Serves 2

In Spain, tortillas are round, flat omelets containing potatoes and onions. Potatoes are a low-calorie, high-fiber food that offers protection against cardiovascular disease and cancer. Meanwhile, onions have the greatest abundance of the inflammation-lowering bioflavanoid quercetin.

8 ounces boiling potatoes
Salt to taste
1 tablespoon ground cumin
1 small zucchini
1 red bell pepper
1 small leek
2 tablespoons olive oil
1 red chile
1 small clove garlic
4 eggs
Black pepper to taste

Wash the potatoes and boil them in salted water with the cumin for about 20 minutes, until tender. Drain, cool, peel, and then cut into thick slices.

Wash, halve lengthwise, and slice the zucchini. Wash and halve the bell pepper, remove seeds and ribs, and chop. Trim off the leek's root and dark green leaves and halve it lengthwise. Wash it well and cut into thin slices.

Heat the oil in a large, nonstick skillet over medium-high heat. Add the potatoes and sauté until golden brown. Add the zucchini, bell pepper, and leek, and sauté over low heat about 5 minutes, stirring gently.

Slit open the chile, remove the seeds, and finely chop the flesh. Peel and mince the garlic. Whisk the chile and garlic with the eggs and season with salt and pepper. Pour the egg mixture over the potatoes and vegetables in the skillet. Cover and cook over very low heat for about 5 minutes, until the eggs are set. With the aid of a rubber spatula, invert the omelet onto a cutting board and slice into wedges to serve.

Whole-Grain Bread with Very Berry Jam Serves 2

Whole grains help lower your cholesterol level, stabilize blood sugar, eliminate sugar cravings, and stabilize levels of serotonin (a chemical messenger in your brain that helps to calm and relax you).

  2 small glass canning jars with screw tops
  9 ounces mixed ripe berries
  4 ounces xylitol, plus more to taste
  1 teaspoon granulated ascorbic acid (natural foods store)
  ½ teaspoon agar-agar (sea vegetable-based gelling agent; Asian market or natural foods store)
  2 tablespoons cold water
  2 tablespoons dairy-free cream cheese (e.g., Soya Kaas or Tofutti)
  2 slices whole-grain (other than wheat) bread
  1 sprig fresh mint

Sterilize the jars by boiling them and the lids in water for 5 minutes. Fill them with the below ingredients while the jars are still hot.

Gently rinse, drain, and cut berries into small pieces. Simmer them in a saucepan with the xylitol and ascorbic acid for 5 minutes over low. If the berry mixture is not sweet enough for your taste, add as much as 1 tablespoon more xylitol to the saucepan.

Stir the agar-agar into the cold water, add it to the saucepan, and simmer for another 2–3 minutes over low.

Immediately transfer the berry jam to the glass canning jars, seal tightly, and let cool.

Spread 2 tablespoons of the cream cheese and 2 tablespoons of the jam on each piece of bread. Garnish with the mint. Refrigerate the remaining jam; eat as soon as possible.

Lunch

Cherry Tomato Salad with Artichoke Hearts   Serves 2

The olive oil in this salad's dressing gives your body a dose of EFAs that trigger fat-burning hormones.

1 tablespoon fresh lemon juice
2 small artichokes (about 18 ounces)
1 ½ tablespoons Bragg Liquid Aminos
Herb salt to taste
Black pepper to taste
2 tablespoons olive oil
1 teaspoon canola oil
1 teaspoon sunflower oil
1 shallot
1 clove garlic
8 ounces cherry tomatoes
½ teaspoon dried dill weed
2 tablespoons chopped fresh Italian parsley
Salt to taste

Add the lemon juice to a medium bowl of water. Snap or slice off the artichoke stems. Scissor off the tough, thorny tips. Pull out the inner leaves and spoon the fuzzy center out of the heart. Put the hearts in the lemon water.

Make the dressing by whisking together the Bragg's, herb salt, and pepper. Gradually whisk in the oils.

Drain the artichoke hearts, slice them into very thin strips, and mix them with the dressing.

Next, peel and dice the shallot and garlic. Rinse and dry the tomatoes, halving larger ones. Add the shallot, garlic, tomatoes, dill weed, and parsley to the artichokes and dressing and toss well. Season with salt and pepper and serve.

Chicken Kabobs with Radi-Cumber Salad   Serves 2

Chicken contains L-tyrosine, which helps your body produce thyroid hormones that drive your metabolism and help to burn calories and regulate your weight more efficiently. It is also a good source of selenium, another key component of thyroid hormone metabolism.

2 wooden skewers (9-inches each)
8 ounces boneless, skinless chicken breast
1 tablespoon lemon juice
Salt to taste
Black pepper to taste
2 tablespoons olive oil
9 ounces cucumber
9 ounces radishes
1 ½ tablespoons Bragg Liquid Aminos
1 teaspoon crushed red pepper flakes
½ teaspoon chopped dill weed
2 tablespoons chopped fresh Italian parsley

Soak skewers in water for 30 minutes. Cube the chicken breast and thread the cubes onto the skewers.

In a shallow dish, mix lemon juice, salt, pepper, and 1/2 tablespoon of the oil. Put the chicken skewers in the marinade and turn to coat. Peel the cucumber, wash the radishes, and cut them into round slices. Broil the skewers for 8–10 minutes in the oven. Meanwhile, stir together Bragg Liquid Aminos, remaining 1 ½ tablespoons olive oil, salt, pepper, red pepper flakes, and the dill weed. Add the cucumber, radishes, and parsley, and toss.

Serve the broiled chicken skewers with the salad.

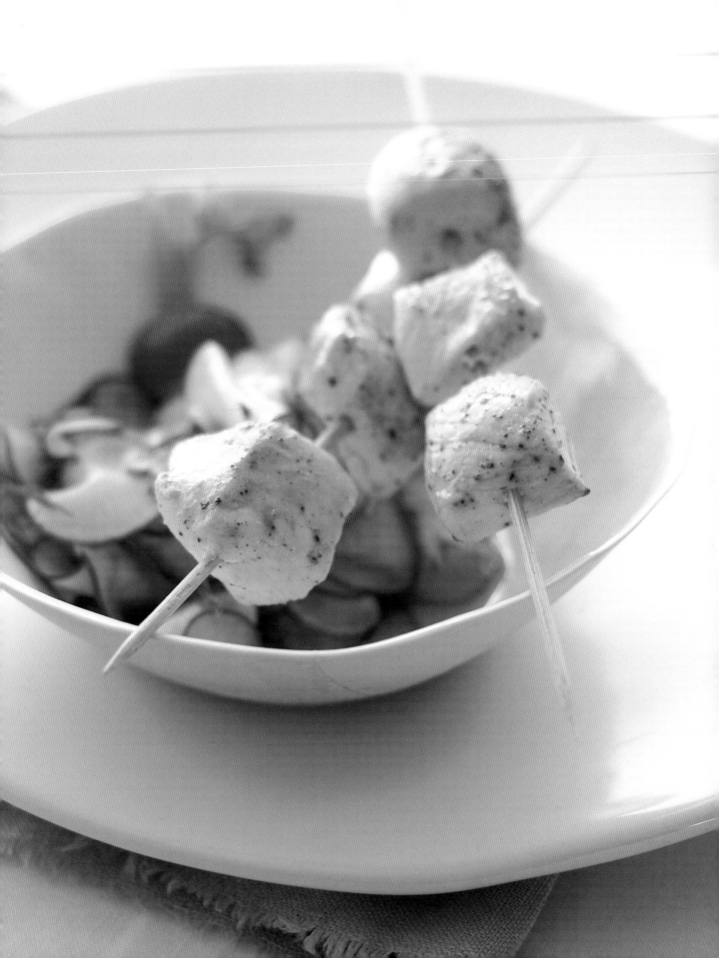

Gazpacho   Serves 4

If you have not yet reached menopause, then you should make tomatoes your close and personal friends. Tomatoes are rich in lycopene, which has been found to significantly reduce the risk of ovarian cancer in premenopausal women.

6 plum tomatoes
½ medium cucumber
½ red bell pepper
½ green bell pepper
1 small red onion
3 cloves garlic
1 ½ cups vegetable juice
Juice of ½ lemon
1 teaspoon Worcestershire sauce
1 tablespoon olive oil
1 tablespoon fresh herbs (e.g., parsley and/or basil; optional)
Salt and pepper to taste

Peel, seed, and dice the tomatoes and cucumber. Dice the bell pepper, onion, and garlic.

In a large bowl, combine all ingredients except the fresh herbs. Refrigerate for 6–8 hours.

Serve chilled, topped with chopped fresh herbs, if desired, and salt and pepper to taste.

Miso Soup   Serves 4

Research shows that regular intake of soy protein, from foods such as tofu and miso, can help you lower total cholesterol levels by as much as 30 percent, lower triglyceride levels, and reduce the tendency of platelets to form blood clots.

    4 dried shiitake or other wild mushrooms
    1 ½ cups boiling water
    2 medium carrots
    2 stalks celery
    4 cups vegetable stock
    1 ½ cups shredded cabbage
    4 tablespoons white miso
    1 cake tofu
    ½ cup sweet corn
    1 sheet nori (seaweed)
    1–2 green onions

Cover the shiitakes with the boiling water in a heatproof bowl. Let sit 10 minutes.

Wash, peel, and slice the carrots diagonally into ¼-inch-thick medallions. Rinse and slice the celery diagonally into ¼-inch-thick crescents.

In a soup pot, cover the carrots and celery with 3 ½ cups of stock and bring to boil. Lower heat and simmer about 10 minutes, until carrots are crisp-tender.

Drain the mushrooms, retaining their soaking liquid to add to the vegetables and stock. Slice the mushroom caps into thin strips and add them to the soup. Stir in the shredded cabbage; simmer until tender but still crunchy.

Stir the miso with the remaining ½ cup of stock in a small bowl. Cube the tofu and add it, with the miso mixture and corn, to the soup. Heat gently, without allowing soup to boil. Toast nori by passing the sheet of seaweed over a gas flame briefly, then crumble it into flakes. Rinse, pat dry, and chop the green onions. Sprinkle green onions and crumbled nori over the top of the soup.

Quesadillas With Salsa   Serves 4

Peppers' vitamin C and bioflavonoids work in concert to protect against heavy menstrual bleeding and free-radical damage.

Quesadillas

1 tablespoon olive oil
1 ½ teaspoons bottled minced garlic
2 cups chopped green bell peppers
½ cup chopped fresh cilantro
1 can black beans (15 ounces), drained and rinsed
4 spelt flour tortillas (8-inches each)
Olive or canola oil cooking spray
¾ cup shredded dairy-free cheese (3 ounces)

Salsa

1 cup corn
½ cup chopped fresh cilantro
1 tablespoon fresh lime juice
1 tablespoon Bragg Liquid Aminos
½ teaspoon minced garlic
1 red bell pepper, chopped

To make the quesadillas, preheat the broiler. Heat olive oil in a large skillet over medium-high heat. Add garlic; sauté 30 seconds. Add green peppers, cilantro, and black beans; cook 5 minutes or until liquid cooks off, stirring occasionally.

Spray a baking sheet with oil and lay tortillas on top. Spoon onto each tortilla ½ cup of bean mixture and 3 tablespoons of cheese; fold in half. Lightly coat tops with cooking spray. Broil 3 minutes or until cheese melts and tortillas begin to brown. Cut each tortilla into three wedges.

For the salsa, mix corn and remaining ingredients in a small saucepan. Bring to boil over high heat; cook for 2 minutes, stirring frequently. Serve with quesadillas.

Svelte Waldorf Salad   Serves 2

This is a lighter version of the salad created at the Waldorf-Astoria Hotel in New York City in the 1890s. Apple pectin has a positive effect on blood glucose levels. And the more stable your blood glucose level, the less likely you are to overeat.

1 egg yolk (the fresher the better)
2 teaspoons fresh lemon juice with pulp
2–3 tablespoons canola oil
¼ cup soy yogurt
Salt to taste
Black pepper to taste
2 ribs celery with leaves
1–2 tart apples
1 ounce pecans, coarsely chopped

Whisk the egg yolk and lemon juice, then slowly whisk in the oil, drop-by-drop. Stir in the yogurt and season with salt and pepper. Rinse and trim the celery, reserving the leaves and slicing the ribs. Wash and core the apples and chop them into ½–¾-inch dice.

Toss all ingredients with the dressing. Season if necessary, sprinkle with pecans, and serve with celery leaf garnish.

Tex-Mex Red Bean Salad   Serves 2

Fiber all-stars, red kidney beans are an excellent source of the trace mineral, molybdenum, which helps your body detoxify sulfites. Plus, their high fiber content prevents blood sugar levels from rising too rapidly after a meal.

4 ounces canned red kidney beans, drained
1 yellow bell pepper
1 avocado
1 teaspoon lemon juice
1 stalk celery
1 small red onion
2 tablespoons Bragg Liquid Aminos
⅛ teaspoon cumin
Salt to taste
Black pepper to taste
Tabasco sauce to taste
3 tablespoons extra virgin olive oil
¼ bunch fresh cilantro
6 leaves butterhead lettuce

Rinse and drain the beans. Wash and core the bell pepper and remove its seeds. Slice the bell pepper into strips. Halve the avocado, cut flesh into narrow wedges, and immediately sprinkle with lemon juice. Wash and trim the celery and thinly slice on the diagonal. Skin and halve the onion, then slice it into half-rings.

Make the dressing by whisking together the Bragg's, cumin, salt, pepper, Tabasco, and oil in a medium bowl. Wash and shake dry the cilantro, chop it, and add it to the dressing. Mix the avocado and vegetables with the dressing.

Gently wash and shake dry the lettuce and arrange three leaves "cup" sides up on each serving plate. Spoon out equal portions of the salad into the lettuce cups.

Turkey with Marinated Asparagus   Serves 2

Just one serving of asparagus supplies almost 60 percent of the daily recommended intake of folic acid.

18 ounces asparagus
Salt to taste
2 teaspoons chopped hazelnuts
1 tablespoon lemon juice
2 tablespoons Bragg Liquid Aminos
Black pepper to taste
2 tablespoons extra virgin olive oil
1 hard-boiled egg
4 ounces red or orange bell pepper
8 leaves fresh basil
2 ounces sliced smoked turkey breast

Rinse the asparagus, snap off the tough ends, and peel the bottom third of the spears. In a saucepan, bring a large quantity of salted water to boil. Add the asparagus spears, cover, reduce heat, and simmer until crisp-tender, about 10–12 minutes.

In an ungreased skillet, toast the hazelnuts until golden brown.

Drain the asparagus, reserving ¼ cup of the cooking water. Make the marinade by whisking together the cooking water, lemon juice, Bragg's, salt, pepper, and oil. Pour the marinade over the asparagus in a shallow dish and refrigerate covered for 2–3 hours.

Shell the egg and slice into eight wedges. Rinse, dry, and slice the bell pepper into thin slivers. Rinse, shake dry, and chop the basil coarsely.

Arrange the egg wedges, bell pepper slivers, and sliced turkey next to the asparagus on serving plates. Sprinkle with the toasted hazelnuts and basil.

Dinner

Asian Chicken and Brown Rice   Serves 4

Brown rice is high in the mineral chromium, which has been shown to help increase lean body mass and decrease the percentage of body fat—both factors in weight loss.

2 tablespoons white miso
1 ½ tablespoons minced ginger
2 garlic cloves, minced
4 skinless, boneless chicken breast
  halves (4 ounces each)
Canola oil spray
5 large egg whites, lightly beaten
1 cup finely chopped onion
1 cup sliced carrot

1 tablespoon fish sauce
2 tablespoons chopped fresh parsley
2 tablespoons chopped green onions
1 cup diced shiitake mushroom caps (about 3 ounces)
2 ½ cups cooked brown rice
1 tablespoon low-sodium soy sauce
1 ½ cups chopped spinach

Combine first three ingredients in a small bowl. Rinse and pat dry chicken breast halves and rub miso mixture over both sides of them. Wrap each breast half securely in plastic wrap. Arrange the packets in steamer rack in a Dutch oven or soup pot. Steam packets, covered, 20 minutes or until done. Remove packets from steamer; let stand 5 minutes. Remove chicken from plastic, reserving liquid from packets. Dice chicken; set aside. Discard water in pan; wipe pan dry with a paper towel.

Place a large, nonstick skillet coated with cooking spray over medium-high heat, when hot, add egg whites and cook 2 minutes or until done. Transfer egg whites from skillet to chopping block; coarsely chop.

Peel and finely chop onion; peel and slice carrot on the diagonal into 1/8-inch-thick ovals. Add reserved cooking packet liquid, chicken, onion, carrot, and fish sauce to Dutch oven, and bring to a boil. Reduce heat to medium; cook 5 minutes or until liquid almost evaporates. Wash, shake dry, and chop the parsley; rinse, pat dry, and slice the green onions and mushroom caps. Add rice, mushrooms, parsley, green onions, and soy sauce to Dutch oven; cook 3 minutes. Stir in egg whites and spinach.

Serve in bowls with chopsticks and/or soup spoons.

Fettuccine Alfredo Serves 8

Once a staple on U.S. Naval ships, navy beans are a good source of cholesterol-lowering fiber. In addition to lowering cholesterol, white beans' high fiber content prevents blood sugar levels from rising too rapidly after a meal.

1 ½ cups corn
1 ½ cups rice milk
1 tablespoon onion powder
1 can navy beans (15.5 ounces), rinsed and drained
1 pound spinach fettuccine
Cracked black pepper

Place corn, milk, and onion powder in a food processor or blender, and process until completely smooth. Pour the blended mixture in a medium saucepan and stir in the beans. Warm over medium-low until the beans are heated through, stirring often.

While sauce is heating, cook the fettuccine in a large pot of boiling water until al dente. Drain well and return pasta to the pot. Add the heated sauce to the pot and toss until evenly coated.

Serve immediately, topping each portion with a generous amount of cracked pepper.

Garbanzo Shepherd's Pie   Serves 6–8

Garbanzos are excellent sources of low-fat protein, fiber, and complex carbohydrates.

4 large potatoes, diced
3 cups rice milk
¼ teaspoon onion powder
1 large onion, chopped
½ pound mushrooms, chopped
½ cup water
1 ½ cups diced carrots
¾ cup diced celery
2 cups spinach leaves
1 tablespoon tamari
½ tablespoon seasoning blend (e.g., Mrs. Dash)
¼ teaspoon garlic powder
2 teaspoons cornstarch, mixed
¼ cup cold water
2 cups garbanzo beans
1 ½ cups frozen peas, thawed
Paprika

Scrub, dice, and steam potatoes over boiling water for 15 minutes. Place in a bowl; add 1 cup rice milk and the onion powder. Mash until smooth.

Preheat oven to 325°F.

Peel and chop onion; and rinse, pat dry, and chop mushrooms. Place the onion and mushrooms in a large pot with the water. Cook, stirring, for 5 minutes. Wash, peel, and dice the carrot and celery; add them to the pot and continue to cook, stirring frequently, until the carrot and celery are tender, about 10 minutes. Add the spinach, cover, and steam until wilted, about 1 minute. Remove from heat.

In a separate saucepan, mix remaining 2 cups of the rice milk with the rice sauce, seasoning blend, and garlic powder. Mix the cornstarch with ¼ cup cold water, and add mixture to saucepan. Cook, stirring, until the mixture boils and thickens. Add to the vegetable mixture, then stir in the garbanzos and peas.

Spoon into six to eight individual casserole dishes. Top with mashed potatoes and sprinkle with paprika. Bake for 30 minutes or until golden.

Hawaiian Grilled Salmon Salad with Tropical Fruit Salsa   Serves 6

Leaf lettuce is rich in lutein and zeaxanthin, two powerful carotenoids that have been associated with reducing your risk for cataracts and macular degeneration.

2 teaspoons olive oil
2 teaspoons lemon juice
1 teaspoon freshly grated ginger
6 salmon fillets (6 ounces each)
6 cups torn fresh leaf lettuce

Combine oil, lemon juice, and ginger and coat both sides of fish. Refrigerate for up to an hour.

Preheat broiler. Place fish fillets under broiler and cook 3–5 minutes or until heated thoroughly.

Divide lettuce among six plates and place a grilled salmon fillet on each. Top with Tropical Fruit Salsa (see page 103 in Snacks & Appetizers section).

Saturated Fats

A diet high in saturated fats has additional risks for women. It increases the likelihood of menstrual cramps, PMS, ovarian cysts, benign breast disease, endometriosis, fibroid tumors, heavy menstrual bleeding, and other female health problems. One reason is that meat and dairy products are the main dietary sources of arachidonic acid, the fat your body uses to produce series-2 prostaglandin hormones, or the "bad" prostaglandins. Regular use of dairy, red meat, and eggs also increases your estrogen level, which can make numerous health conditions worse, including many of the reproductive conditions listed above.

Tips:
→ Replace potato chips and corn chips with either unsalted hard pretzels or low-salt, baked chips.
→ Use safflower or canola oil-based mayonnaise.
→ Try a garden burger or veggie dog instead of a hamburger or hotdog at your next cookout.

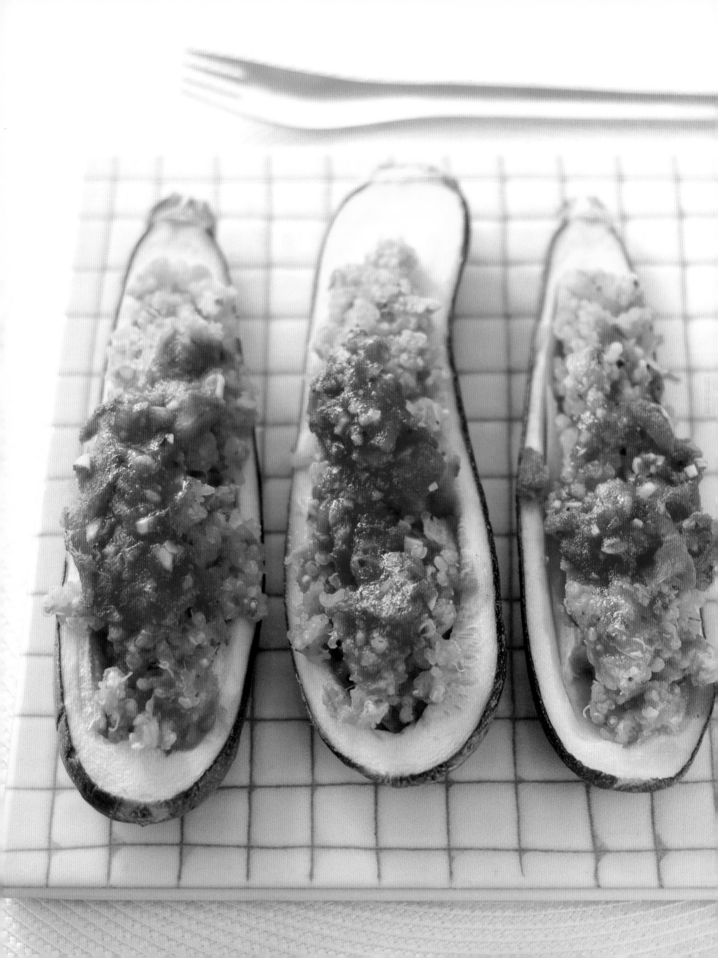

Quinoa-Stuffed Zucchini   Serves 2

Quinoa contains more protein than any other grain, and is considered a complete protein due to the fact that is contains all eight essential amino acids.

2 large zucchini
1 onion, chopped
1 tablespoon olive oil
1 teaspoon dried marjoram
½ teaspoon basil
2 carrots, grated
½ cup red lentils
3 cups water
1 cup uncooked quinoa
Salt and pepper to taste
1 can crushed tomatoes
5 cloves crushed garlic
1 teaspoon chili powder
2 teaspoons seasoning blend (e.g., Mrs. Dash)

Halve zucchinis and scoop out their centers, leaving the shells. Peel and chop the onion, as well as the zucchini flesh. Heat oil in a large skillet. Add onion, zucchini flesh, marjoram, and basil. Sauté until tender.

Wash, peel, and grate carrots. In a separate pot, combine carrots, lentils, and water. Simmer for about 15 minutes, then add quinoa, lower heat, and let simmer, covered, for 10–15 minutes. Remove from heat and let stand covered for another 10 minutes.

Meanwhile, make a sauce by combining the undrained can of tomatoes and the seasonings.

Stir together the carrot-lentils and the zucchini mixture and spoon into the zucchini shells. Top with tomato sauce. Bake at 350°F for 45 minutes.

Sautéed Shrimp & Vegetables   Serves 2

Shrimp are an excellent source of selenium, a very good source of vitamins D and B12, and an unusually low-fat, low-calorie protein. A four-ounce serving of shrimp supplies 23.7 grams of protein for only 112 calories and less than one gram of fat.

5 ounces sugar snap peas
Salt to taste
1 yellow bell pepper
1 shallot
1 tablespoon canola oil
Black pepper to taste
5 ounces raw, peeled shrimp
4 ounces cherry tomatoes
¼ bunch fresh dill
1 teaspoon toasted caraway seeds
1 tablespoon Bragg Liquid Aminos

Remove any tough parts or strings from the snap peas. Blanch the pods in boiling, salted water for 1 minute, plunge them into cold water, and drain. Wash and quarter the bell pepper; remove its stem, ribs, and seeds, and cut it into julienne strips. Peel and mince the shallot.

In a skillet, heat the oil over medium; add the snap peas, bell pepper, and shallot; and sauté for 5 minutes. Season with salt and pepper. Add the shrimp and sauté for 2 minutes over low heat.

Halve the tomatoes; wash, shake dry, and chop the dill, and add both to the skillet to sauté for another 2 minutes. Remove from the stove and toss contents of skillet with Bragg's.

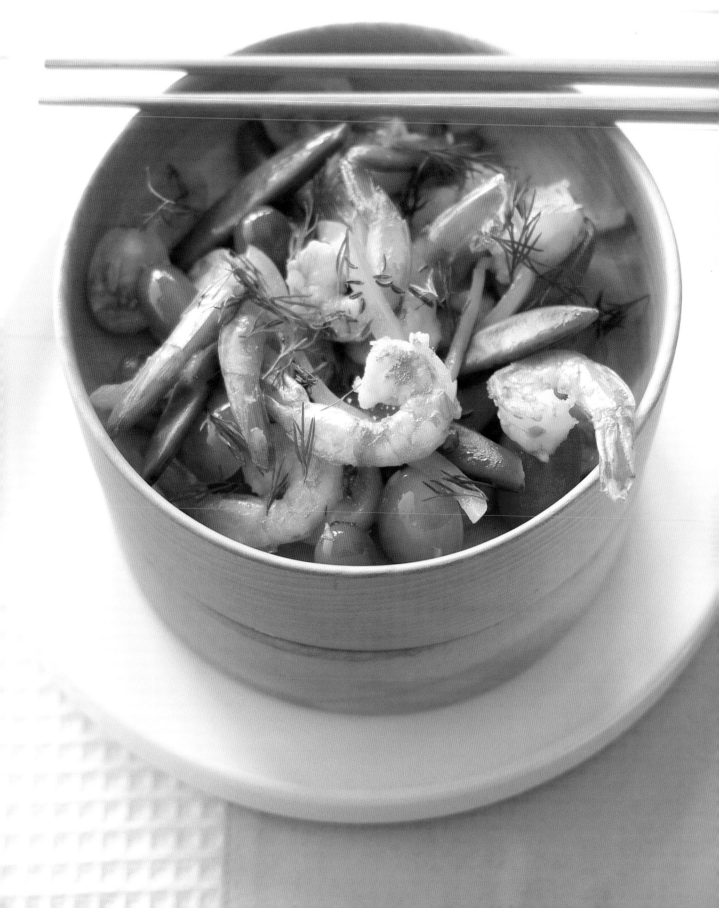

Stir-Fried Garbanzos & Green Veggies Serves 2

Garbanzo beans contain appetite-satisfying L-phenylalanine, an essential amino acid that functions as a natural anti-depressant and improves memory, mood, and libido, as well as boosting your metabolism.

8 ounces spinach leaves
1 green bell pepper
5 ounces green onions
4 ounces sugar snap peas
1 small celery stalk
1 thumbnail-sized piece of fresh ginger
1 clove garlic
1 tablespoon canola oil
9 ounces cooked garbanzo beans, drained
3 ½ tablespoons vegetable stock
Salt to taste
Cayenne pepper to taste
1–2 teaspoons lemon juice
2 tablespoons soy yogurt

Thoroughly wash and stem the spinach and chop it coarsely. Wash and quarter the bell pepper; remove its stem, ribs, and seeds, and cut it into julienne strips. Cut washed and trimmed green onions diagonally into pieces. Remove any tough parts or strings from the peas. Wash and trim celery stalk and cut diagonally into bite-sized pieces. Peel ginger and garlic and mince.

In a wok or skillet, heat the oil over high and briefly stir-fry the ginger and garlic in it. Add the julienned bell pepper, the peas, celery, and green onions, and sauté for about 4 minutes, stirring constantly.

Add the spinach, garbanzos, and stock and sauté for another 2–3 minutes. Season to taste with salt, cayenne, and lemon juice. Spoon even portions onto plates and dollop 1 tablespoon of yogurt in the center of each serving.

Thai Tilapia Serves 4

A staple food fish in Africa, tilapia features low-fat flesh that is sweet and fine-textured, and is an excellent substitute in recipes for many kinds of fish, including sole, snapper, pompano, flounder, cod, sea bass, and orange roughy

2 teaspoons sesame oil
2 garlic cloves, minced
2 teaspoons peeled, minced fresh ginger
1 cup chopped red bell pepper
1 cup chopped shallots
2 teaspoons curry powder
½ teaspoon ground cumin
4 teaspoons tamari sauce
1 tablespoon xylitol
14 ounces coconut milk
2 tablespoons chopped fresh cilantro
4 tilapia fillets (6 ounces each)
Olive oil
3 teaspoons sesame seeds
2 cups cooked basmati rice

Preheat broiler.

Heat 1 teaspoon of sesame oil over medium-high heat. Add garlic and ginger and cook for 1–2 minutes, until fragrant. Add bell pepper and shallots and cook 2 minutes. Stir in curry powder and cumin and cook 1 minute. Add tamari, xylitol, and coconut milk and bring to a simmer. Add cilantro and immediately remove from heat.

Brush fish with remaining 1 teaspoon of sesame oil and sprinkle with sesame seeds. Place on broiler pan brushed with olive oil and broil for 8 minutes (or until fish flakes easily). Place fish on top of rice and top with sauce. Serve hot.

Dessert

Apple-Cinnamon Quinoa "Cake" Makes 1 cake

Once called "the gold of the Incas," quinoa supplies complete protein. Commonly referred to as a "grain," quinoa is actually related to leafy, green veggies, like spinach and Swiss chard.

2 cups organic apple juice
1 cup water
1 pinch sea salt
1 ¼ cups quinoa
1 teaspoon ground cinnamon
½ teaspoon vanilla

Bring water and apple juice to a boil with a pinch of salt. Add quinoa and cinnamon. Stir and cook on low for 10–15 minutes, until all liquid is absorbed. Remove from heat and stir in vanilla. Let sit 10 minutes.

Rinse an 8- x 8-inch baking dish; do not dry. Pack quinoa into the baking dish. Allow to cool before cutting into squares or dishing into balls with an ice cream scoop.

Refined Sugar

While you cannot control the amount of sugar that is automatically added to many foods, you can manage your intake by monitoring labels and refraining from adding sugar to foods such as cereal, oatmeal, homemade sweets, and tea. I advise against using artificial sweeteners in place of refined sugar. They have no nutritional value and may worsen PMS and general anxiety symptoms.

Tips:
→ Try honey instead of sugar in your tea.
→ When baking desserts, try maple syrup.
→ Mix applesauce and raisins into your oatmeal.
→ Attack those sweet cravings with a bowl of fresh fruit topped with a spoonful of vanilla soy yogurt.

Chilled Fruit Soup   Serves 8

Cantaloupe derives its name from the Italian village of Cantalup, where it was first cultivated around 1700 A.D. The extremely sweet and juicy melon is also extremely well endowed with vitamins A and C.

1 ripe cantaloupe (about 2 cups melon balls or bite-sized chunks)
1 ripe banana, peeled
4 large, ripe peaches, pitted
5 cups pineapple juice
2 cups fresh blueberries
¼ teaspoon freshly grated nutmeg
¼ teaspoon cinnamon
1 cup ice cubes
1 tablespoon fresh lemon juice
1 teaspoon vanilla
Mint sprigs for garnish

Blend cantaloupe in food processor or blender. Add banana, peaches, and 2 cups pineapple juice. Purée till smooth. Pour into a large pitcher or punchbowl.

Purée 1 cup berries with spices, ice cubes, lemon juice, and remaining pineapple juice until smooth. Stir berry and cantaloupe mixtures together in a pitcher or punchbowl, adding the remaining berries. Chill at least 1 hour.

Ladle into bowls and garnish with mint.

Baked Pears   Serves 4

Juicy, flavorful pears are a hypoallergenic fruit with high fiber content.

    4 large pears, peeled, cored, and quartered
    ½ cup apple juice
    1 teaspoon ground nutmeg
    1 teaspoon ground cinnamon
    4 teaspoons chopped walnuts

Preheat oven to 350°F.

Core pears and place in a baking dish with the apple juice. Sprinkle with nutmeg and cinnamon. Cover baking dish with foil. Bake for 30 minutes.

Meanwhile, toast walnuts in a single layer on an ungreased baking sheet at 350°F for 5 minutes or until nuts are fragrant and lightly browned. Sprinkle toasted walnuts into hollow cores and on top of baked pears and serve.

Blackberry Sorbet   Serves 2

A wonderful source of vitamin A, potassium, calcium, and magnesium, berries offer so many health benefits.

    9 ounces fresh blackberries
    2 teaspoons lime juice
    1 tablespoon maple syrup
    ¼ cup water
    Dash of vanilla
    1 sprig fresh mint

Gently wash and drain the berries. Set a few aside for garnish.

Purée the remaining berries with the lime juice, maple syrup, water, and vanilla. Transfer the purée to a stainless steel bowl, cover, and freeze 3–4 hours, stirring every hour.

Spoon the sorbet into dessert bowls, garnish with berries and mint and enjoy.

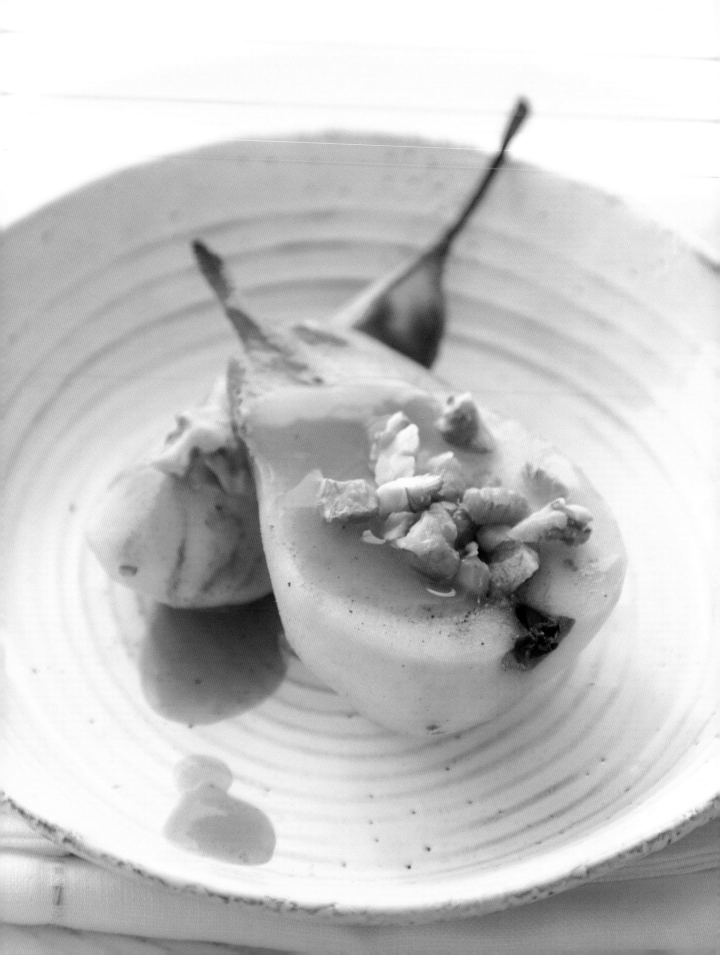

Pumpkin Oatmeal Cookies   Makes 4–5 dozen cookies

If you are overly acidic, you should eat five to seven servings a day of grains such as oats. If you are a high alkaline producer, we recommend one to two servings of grains. Pumpkin provides an added shot of vitamins A and C, potassium, dietary fiber, and manganese.

1 cup canned or cooked pumpkin
¾–1 cup xylitol (about 7 ounces)
2 eggs
1 teaspoon vanilla
3 cups rolled oats
1 ½ cups rice flour
1 teaspoon baking soda
1 teaspoon baking powder
1 teaspoon cinnamon
½ teaspoon nutmeg
½ teaspoon ground cloves
1 cup raisins
Canola oil spray (if necessary)

Heat oven to 350°F.

In the bowl of an electric mixer fitted with the paddle attachment, cream pumpkin and xylitol on medium speed until light and fluffy, about 3 minutes. Add eggs; mix on high speed to combine. Mix in vanilla; set aside.

Combine oats, rice flour, baking soda, and baking powder in a large bowl. Stir to combine. Add the flour mixture to the pumpkin mixture, and beat on low speed to combine, 10–15 seconds. Remove bowl from mixer, and stir in spices and raisins.

Drop by spoonfuls on non-stick or oil-sprayed cookie sheets, about 2 inches apart. Bake until golden and just set, about 18 minutes. Transfer cookies to wire rack to cool.

Papaya Soup   Serves 4

This sweet soup has the benefits of papaya's digestive enzyme, papain; soy foods' metabolism-driving L-tyrosine amino acid; and honey's anti-viral, free-radical-fighting properties.

4 cups peeled, chopped papaya (about 2 medium papayas)
2 teaspoons orange juice
1 cup dairy-free sour cream
½ teaspoon vanilla
1 cup rice or soy milk
¼ cup honey
4 strawberries or mint sprigs for garnish

Peel, deseed, and chop papaya; then blend papaya, orange juice, sour cream, vanilla, rice or soy milk, and honey in a blender until smooth. Chill for 1–4 hours.

Garnish with mint leaves or sliced strawberries and serve.

Strawberries with Chocolate & Vanilla Dips   Serves 2

The Aztecs cultivated the vanilla bean, the fruit of a celadon-colored orchid. Once considered an aphrodisiac, vanilla rouses your kidneys, fortifies your stomach, and promotes proper digestion.

9 ounces fresh strawberries
1 ½ ounces Dagoba or other high-quality organic, dark chocolate
¼ cup almond milk
½ vanilla bean
1 teaspoon floral honey
¼ cup vanilla soy yogurt

Gently rinse and dry the strawberries. To make the chocolate dip, coarsely chop the chocolate and put it in a bowl with 3 tablespoons of the almond milk. Melt the chocolate in a hot-but-not-boiling double boiler over low heat, stirring constantly. Let the chocolate dip cool.

To make the vanilla dip, slit the vanilla bean lengthwise, remove the seeds with a paring knife, and mix them with the honey, the remaining 1 tablespoon almond milk, and the vanilla soy yogurt.

Dip the strawberries into the chocolate and vanilla mixtures and enjoy.

The ABCs of Super Health and Glowing Beauty

Apple

A 1978 study showed that apple pectin has a positive effect on blood glucose levels. And the more stable your blood glucose level, the less likely you are to overeat.

Plus, apples are high in quercetin, a bioflavonoid found to be highly effective in lowering inflammation and inhibiting the release of histamines and other inflammatory substances.

Dark Chocolate

While I haven't been a huge fan of chocolate in the past, recent research has made me give pause. According to the April 2000 issue of *Internal Medicine News*, chocolate and cocoa do provide some sound health benefits, including heart protection. Researchers found that dark chocolate is rich in antioxidants, particularly polyphenols and quercetin.

So, if you need to feed your soul, I suggest induling in high quality, organic dark chocolate from Dagoba. Available in most Whole Food Market stores, or at *www.healthyshopping.com*.

Edamame

Edamame—or soybeans—are particularly beneficial for women approaching or experiencing menopause. These foods are rich in isoflavones, a weak estrogenic substance that binds to the estrogen receptors on tissues throughout your body. In perimenopause, isoflavones take the edge off of estrogen dominance by making it harder for your body's own, more potent estrogen to bind to the receptors. In menopause, isoflavones occupy vacant receptor sites and bolster the action of the estrogen your body is still producing.

Flaxseed

If I were stranded on a desert island and could have only one food with me, I'd pick flax. Rich in fiber as well as crucial omega-3 and omega-6 essential fatty acids, just one serving of flax promotes good heart health, helps support normal cholesterol levels, supports healthy joints and strong bones, as well as healthy breast tissue, and supports our immune system and cellular health. Flax also promotes proper sugar metabolism and healthy skin. Plus, it helps you in your weight loss efforts by creating a feeling of "fullness," thanks to its high fiber content.

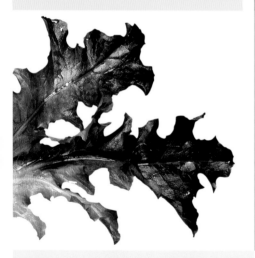

Hummus

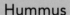

Hummus consists of puréed garbanzo beans, which are excellent sources of low-fat protein, fiber, and complex carbohydrates. Hummus is also rich in the B vitamins essential for regulation of hormone levels and critical to just about every body function. Combine your hummus with whole grains and green, leafy vegetables, and you help ensure that your body gets the essential fatty acids it need to produce inflammation-fighting, series 3 prostaglandins–substances that help prevent PMS symptoms, menstrual cramps, and a host of other female-related troubles.

Iced Green Tea

Several studies have indicated that green tea may prevent certain diseases, thanks to its high concentration of polyphenols, antioxidants that confer even greater protection than vitamins C and E. Polyphenols appear to enhance the activity of your body's antioxidant and detoxifying enzymes, including such key enzymes as glutathione peroxidase and glutathione S-transferase.

Leaf Lettuce

Leaf lettuce is rich in lutein and zeaxanthin, two powerful carotenoids that have been associated with reducing your risk for cataracts and. A landmark study published in the November 1994 issue of the *Journal of the American Medical Association* found that increased intake of the carotenoids lutein and zeaxanthin was strongly associated with a decreased risk for age-related macular degeneration. They found that green leafy vegetables were particularly effective.

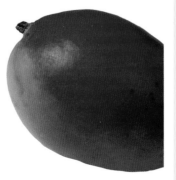

Mangos

Mangos are rich in folic acid, which is necessary for the production of healthy red blood cells and helps prevent cervical dysplasia, a condition that can be a precursor to cancer of the cervix. Folic acid also supports the adrenal glands to enhance energy and stamina, supports normal cholesterol levels, and supports the health of the brain and nervous system in the body.

Broccoli

Broccoli is rich in dindolylmethane (DIM), a plant compound associated with lowering a woman's risk of breast cancer. A 2001 study looked at the dietary habits of postmeno pausal Swedish women aged 50–74. On average they consumed a wide variety of foods, including 19 different commonly eaten fruits and vegetables. Researchers found that those women who ate 1–2 servings of Brassica foods a day had a 20–40 percent lower risk of breast cancer than those women who ate virtually none.

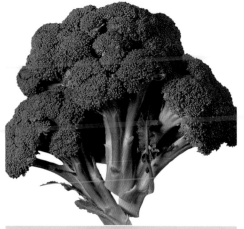

Carrots

In addition to being rich in vitamin A, carrots are high in alpha-carotene, an antioxidant found to significantly reduce the risk of the disease in post-menopausal women.

Plus, animal studies have shown that alpha-carotene is 10 times more effective than beta-carotene in suppressing lung, liver, and skin cancer, while other research has found that the nutrient is 38 percent stronger in antioxidant activity than beta-carotene.

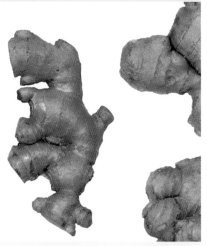

Ginger

One of the most effective remedies for nausea is ginger. On another note, ginger has been used as an aphrodisiac for centuries. Even today, women in Senegal wear ginger in their belts in order to attract men, while female New Guineans can't say no to a man who emits ginger's strong scent.

To make your own tea, cut fresh ginger into small pieces and steep in boiling hot water for about 25 minutes.

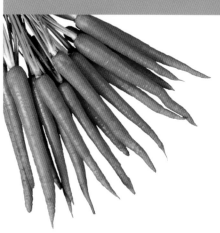

Juicy Melons

In addition to being high in beta-carotene and vitamin C, melons provide a healthy, alkaline alternative to sugar-laden treats. Watermelon is particularly beneficial for women, as it contains lycopene, a carotenoid that has been associated with lowering a woman's risk for female-related cancers.

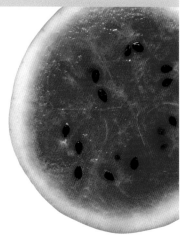
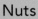

Kava

Pacific Islanders have used kava for centuries to relieve pain and promote relaxation both general and muscular). A potent sedative and anti-anxiety herb, kava is also used to relax tense muscles.

I recommend taking 140–210 mg of a standardized extract of kava lactones per day, with meals. If your mouth tingles right after you swallow the kava, don't worry; this is normal. Do not take kava for more than one or two months at a time.

Nuts

Nuts are nature's way of proving that great things do come in small packages. Eaten raw and whole, they are great sources of healthful polyunsaturated fats; the B-complex vitamins; vitamins A, D, and E; and a wealth of minerals, including calcium, potassium, magnesium, iron, copper, zinc, and phosphorous.

Need more reasons to go nuts? These treasures are also an important source of essential fatty acids (EFAs) that your body can't manufacture. The best nut choices are almonds and walnuts.

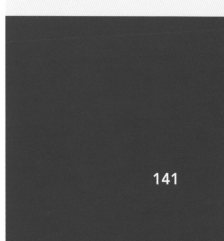

141

Olive Oil

Olive oil is a great source of essential fatty acids (EFAs), fats that your body does not produce and that you must therefore obtain through diet or supplementation. EFAs help to substantially lower your risk of heart disease by lowering LDL cholesterol and triglycerides, preventing blood platelets from becoming sticky, and lowering blood pressure. They also help with bone health, heart health, and depression.

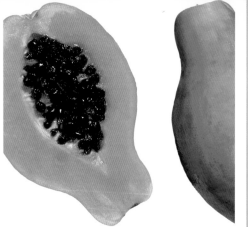

Papaya

Papaya is the perfect food. Naturally alkaline and low in sugar, this fruit is high in both vitamin C and carotenoids, a powerful combination for your skin. For one thing, the two nutrients work together to build and maintain collagen, the protein that gives blood vessels their strength and integrity. Vitamin C does this by assisting the enzymes that participate in collagen production. Carotenoids suppress premenstrual acne and oily skin, and balance your adrenal system. They have even been shown to help to protect your eyesight.

Salmon

Wild salmon is a wonderful source of EFA-packed protein. It contains a complete range of the essential amino acids needed to build protein, and is lower in heart-unhealthy satur-ated fat than red meat or pork. Plus, it's a great source of vitamins A, D, and E.

I recommend eating a four- to six-ounce serving of salmon several times a week. I am partial to SeaBear Salmon (800-260-1620), wild Alaskan salmon that has been carefully tested and is free of harmful contaminants.

Valerian Root

Valerian root, a perennial plant found in North America, Europe, and Asia, was used during World War I to prevent frontline troops from developing shell shock, and during World War II to reduce anxiety among civilians exposed to air raids. Today, valerian root can be taken for depression, stress relief, and insomnia.

If you are having difficulty falling asleep or staying asleep, I have found that valerian root can be very beneficial. Valerian root has also been used to treat fatigue, intestinal cramps and other nervous conditions.

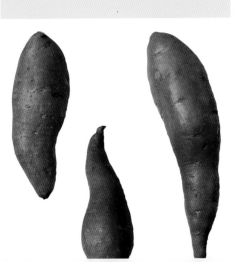

Yams

Like leaf lettuce, yams are rich in lutein and zeaxanthin. Yams are also high in beta-carotene, which helps boost your immune system, improves the health of your skin, suppresses premenstrual acne and oily skin, and balances the adrenal system to enhance energy and stamina. Beta-carotene is also needed for the normal production of red blood cells, helping prevent fatigue caused by anemia or heavy menstrual bleeding.

Quinoa

It is common knowledge that wheat is one of the two most common food allergens, but recent research is finding that wheat intolerance is not only on the rise, it is becoming more serious. According to a February 2003 study from the *Archives of Internal Medicine,* more than 1.5 million Americans have celiac disease, a digestive condition that is triggered by gluten—a protein found in wheat, rye, and barley.

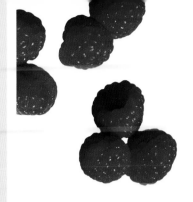

Raspberries

For me, berries are nature's candy. Not only are they sweet and delicious, but they can also help prevent or relieve a wide variety of health complaints. From antioxidants that fight cancer and heart disease, to bioflavonoids and minerals essential for energy and good bones, the nutrients in berries benefit your whole body—and come in a sweet, attractive, richly textured package. A wonderful source of vitamin A, potassium, calcium, and magnesium, berries offer so many health benefits.

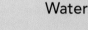

Tomatoes

If you have not yet reached menopause, then you should quickly make tomatoes your close and personal friends. Tomatoes are rich in lycopene, which has been found to significantly reduce the risk of ovarian cancer in premenopausal women. Just be sure to mix the tomatoes in an oil base, such as olive oil, to enhance lycopene absorption in the body.

Unrefined Grains

Whole, unrefined grains have been the mainstay of the human diet and our main source of energy for years. They provide fiber, protein, carbohydrates, fats, B complex and other important vitamins, as well as a wealth of minerals, including calcium, magnesium, potassium, iron, copper, and manganese. They are also excellent sources of lignans (certain chemicals found in plants that mimic the effect of estrogen in women), helping with numerous reproductive problems.

Water

Everything in your body depends on water. In fact, water makes up 82 percent of your blood, 75 percent of your muscle, 25 percent of your bone, 76 percent of your brain tissue, and 90 percent of your lung tissue! Plus, water neutralizes acidity, which can dry out your skin.

Water, whether mineral or distilled, is a great way to detoxify your system, curb hunger, rejuvenate your skin, and oxygenate your body.

Xylitol

Xylitol is a little-known plant sugar that's a far better alternative to refined white sugar and artificial sweeteners. It's completely healthy, with no aftertaste. Xylitol won't raise your blood sugar as fast as regular sugar, and it raises the pH in the mouth, so it helps prevent dental cavities. And it even has one- third fewer calories than regular sugar.

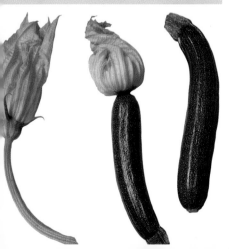

Zucchini

Zucchini consists of more than 95 percent water, which makes it a great, low-calorie vegetable. It is also chock full of fiber, so it helps to fill you up and keep you feeling full—which means fewer hunger pangs for you.

Zucchini is also rich in a wide variety of female-beneficial nutrients, including potassium and phosphorus, both of which help to keep your body in a slightly alkaline state. Plus, these minerals have a powerful effect on your energy production.

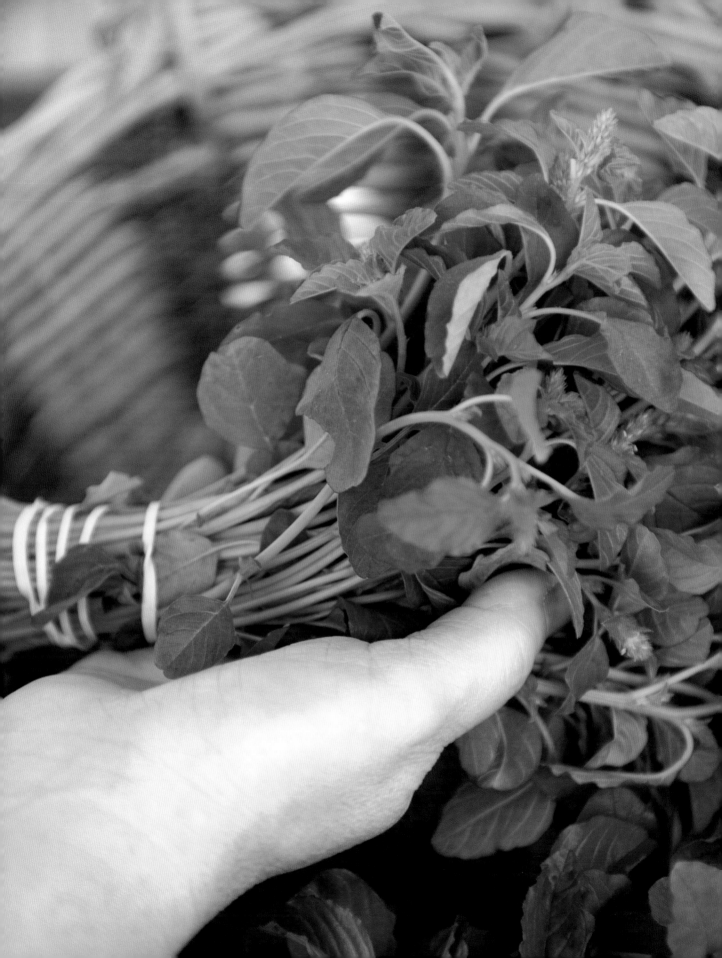

Detox for Life

If you've heard of liver "cleanses" that start off with a three-day fast and end with harsh laxatives and a few rough hours of needing to stay close to the bathroom, let me reassure you, that's not what this chapter is about. Although I do advocate bi-yearly or even quarterly intensive liver-detox programs, I believe it makes more sense for most women to start with a gentler, daily program they can maintain as part of a healthier, liver-friendly lifestyle that constantly nurtures and supports their liver.

Don't mistake "gentle" for "less effective"—this program will begin reaping benefits immediately. And, when more intensive, "purge"-type liver cleanses are done within an already liver-loving daily lifestyle, their effects are less harsh and less likely to cause uncomfortable side effects, because there are fewer toxins to clean out. This is a much healthier and more effective approach than living a liver-abusive lifestyle, then trying to play "catch-up" to redeem liver health with periodic and harsh major cleanses.

Detoxification is one of your liver's most important and vital functions. Because it helps to cleanse and invigorate your cells and tissues, it's a great way to ramp up your ability to lose weight. It also promotes radiant skin and lustrous hair. But more importantly, by eliminating toxins from your body detox protects your nervous system and brain from unmetabolized toxins; reduces your risk of heart disease, PMS, fibroid tumors, endometriosis, and breast cancer; enhances your sexual performance and libido; combats fatigue and low energy; and supports estrogen metabolism.

As your primary organ of detoxification, your liver is a devoted bodyguard. Every day, you're exposed to thousands of substances and other factors that could seriously harm you, and in order to protect you against them, your liver quite literally places itself in harm's way—between you and those toxins. In this chapter, let's take a look at how small changes in what you eat, how you think and feel, and the supplements you take can help you care for your liver—and even rebuild it.

Take Out the Trash

People often think good health is the *absence of disease*—a sort of medical neutral zone. And as evidence of their healthiness, they proudly point out how long it's been since they had a cold or the flu. However, in my experience, truly great health is a far cry from neutral. It's an energetic, luminous state that practically sparkles with vitality. Most people have it when they're too young to appreciate it, then pine for it when they think it's too late to get it back. By middle age, in fact, the absence of disease may seem like a pretty good consolation prize. But you don't have to settle for that.

In most cases, you can have improved health practically overnight, and watch it elevate to great health in a matter of a few months, simply by taking targeted care of the one organ in your body that works tirelessly, every day of your life, to care for you—your liver. Neglect it, and it may continue working hard for you, but "neutral" health will be the best it can deliver. Help it, and it can elevate you to vibrant, brilliant health so vital that you'll be able to feel it, and see it in the mirror. So, as you read this guidebook to the land of Super Health and Glowing Beauty, I'd like you to ask yourself a question: How healthy and toxin-free are *you*?

The Original Multitasker

Your liver has lots of jobs, such as helping you metabolize fats, carbohydrates, and proteins; storing extra blood and key nutrients for use when they're needed; helping manufacture and balance your hormones;

and—as I mentioned earlier—detoxifying and eliminating poisonous wastes and byproducts. This is by far the toughest thing it has to do.

Unfortunately, modern life, which is supposed to have made life easier for all of us, makes things significantly harder for our already hardworking livers. That's because we're practically marinating in toxins our livers were never designed to handle, such as pounds of food additives, preservatives, waxes, coloring agents, industrial and chemical pollutants, drugs, and pesticide and herbicide residues in the food you eat, the air you breathe, and the water you drink. Prescription and over-the counter drugs, traditionally thought of as "beneficial" in one way or another, also put a tremendous toxic burden on your liver. Then there are the toxic fumes leaking from carpets, upholstery, insulation, refrigerators, air conditioners, etc. Plus, myriad substances you create within your own body—such as hormones that must be broken down—are significant lever stressors, including the relentlessly elevated cortisol levels from your own adrenals (thanks to chronic stress). And, those poor food choices I mentioned are not only tough for your liver to metabolize, burdening it with toxic byproducts, but they also provide no real nutrition for your liver to use for needed self-repairs.

And here's an enormous liver burden about which most of us are oblivious: A woman's mind and spirit can add to her liver's toxic load, if her thoughts and feelings are negative. In fact, everything you think, feel, and believe affects the health of your liver and its ability to detoxify and keep your body healthy. The link between your thoughts and emotions and the health of your liver is well known, and well validated by research.

Toxic Backwash

So, now you know what your liver is supposed to do with the toxins that threaten you, and you know that it's overworked. What happens next? It gradually loses its ability to break down and eliminate the toxins your bloodstream constantly delivers to its doorstep. Over time, toxins that are only partially broken down (and thus still somewhat poisonous) begin accumulating in your liver's cells and ductwork, sickening the organ itself, and setting it up for inflammatory disease, such as hepatitis, and the scar tissue that inevitably follows. Stockpiled toxic waste begins spilling out of the liver, and your whole body becomes increasingly toxic, scrambling to eliminate toxins through less efficient, less reliable, secondary routes—for example, excreting still-toxic wastes through the pores of your skin, into your urine, lungs, and intestinal tract.

As a result, your skin becomes more sensitive, more easily inflamed, and increasingly prone to severe sunburn. You may experience increased oiliness, clogged pores, dryness, flakiness, a blotchy, blemished, "ruddy" complexion on your face and other exposed areas, thinned "older-looking" skin, and a tired, sallow appearance. Your lungs may become easier targets for respiratory ailments, sensitivities, and allergies. Your digestive tract may also begin to lose some of its ability to handle food efficiently, leading to indigestion, gas, unexplained weight gain, and a sensitive, overreactive gut that leaves you reluctant to eat anywhere that

doesn't provide easy access to a private bathroom. Plus, your kidneys can become stressed, leading to retained water and bloating, rising blood pressure, and increased vulnerability to vaginal, urinary tract, and kidney infections.

Thanks to all this toxic backwash, you may begin to feel chronically fatigued, prone to headaches, bloated, irritable, emotionally reactive, and mentally foggy—eventually feeling as though you can no longer rely on your body or your mind.

My Love-Your-Liver Program

Now that you understand how important your liver is, and how serious the consequences of neglecting it can be, you can start taking steps to clear out the toxins it has accumulated, as well as those that may have been diverted to your secondary organs of detoxification—your skin, lungs, intestinal tract, and kidneys. Detoxifying your body pulls stashed toxins out of hiding, bringing them into the blood and lymph circulation where they can be properly eliminated.

In the process, their brief presence in your circulation can make you temporarily more toxic—until your detox program successfully eliminates them. This is immediately accompanied by a significant improvement in the way you look and feel, which escalates as your liver repairs and regenerates.

If you feel nervous about detox programs due to a bad experience with other programs that are harsh and difficult to follow, rest assured, this program is different. Even if you believe you are healthy to begin with, you'll see and feel clear evidence of improvement within days to weeks.

With my daily program, you can start slowly and work up, one step at a time, rebuilding and regenerating as you go. That way, you'll cleanse your liver and secondary detox centers, and strengthen and restore your liver's functional capacity to protect you, all at the same time, with less risk of reactions, such as unexplained headaches, fatigue, bad breath, rashes, diarrhea, or flu-like symptoms. My six-step daily detox program, in conjunction with the recipes in this chapter, lets you take it slowly and customize, according to your specific needs. Are you ready to love your liver? The sooner you begin, the sooner you'll see for yourself that this is one of those instances where the love you give comes back to you many-fold.

1. Drink more pure water. If you haven't been diligent about drinking lots of water, now is the time to start. As you liberate stored toxins, it will take plenty of water to flush them safely and completely from your system through every possible route of elimination: Urine, stool, the moisture in exhaled breath, and sweat.

The water you drink should be purified mineral water. Shoot for a minimum of eight 8-ounce glasses a day, evenly spread out over the day, and increase the amount, as necessary, if you engage in any activity that increases your breathing rate or your sweat production. And, if your self assessment from Chapter One indicates that you're overly acidic, take the time to re-read that information now, and learn how to boost your alkalinization by adding supplemental bicarbonate to your water.

2. Increase your intake of healthy, organic foods. By eating the foods featured in the detoxifying recipes at the end of this chapter, you'll be eating a predominantly vegetarian diet, with emphasis on raw and steamed foods. This gives you a nutritional program that is not only delicious, but also centered on healthy, organic whole foods—salads, steamed vegetables, whole grains, legumes, and lots of fiber to help move toxins through your colon, all based on my pH-balance philosophy. Include the specific foods listed on page 152, known in traditional Chinese medicine to specifically and gently cleanse and restore liver function. For animal-based protein, eat eggs prepared without oils (i.e. soft- or hard-boiled), or choose easy-to-digest fish and poultry, such as wild, organic salmon or free-range chicken.

Be sure to make your dietary changes gradually and gently. That way, detox will occur gradually and gently, and the improvement in how you feel will help motivate you to make this your new way of eating for life.

3. Avoid foods that add to your liver's stress load. As I discussed in Chapter One, there are certain categories of foods you should work to reduce, if not eliminate, due to their acidic nature. Interestingly, most of these foods can also generate toxic residues that your liver must neutralize (such as alcohol, red meat, fatty foods, and refined sugar). Others, such as caffeine, over-stimulate your adrenals and increase already chronic secretion of cortisol, for increased nervous tension and the toxic metabolites of breaking down that hormone. Finally, wheat and dairy can trigger inflammatory reactions, increasing your liver's need to detoxify histamines and leukotrienes in your body.

4. Don't eat after 7 PM. Nighttime is your liver's time to regenerate, not to deal with late night meals or snacks. Eat your heaviest meal towards midday, and make your last meal of the day not only earlier than usual, but also lighter.

5. Try a light, modified, one-day fast every three months. If you're working and active, a true fast can be disruptive. However, once you've gotten this far in the program, you may feel up to an intermittent, modified fast, to help boost the clearance of toxins from your liver while maintaining your usual daily routine and avoiding the anxiety that comes with anticipating hunger. To do this, eat two or three light meals a day, consisting of fresh organic vegetable juices (celery, carrot, beet, beet greens, parsley, cucumber, spinach, garlic, and/or wheatgrass), low-fat and low-sodium vegetable broths, herbal teas, uncooked or lightly steamed organic vegetables, and thoroughly cooked organic starches, grains, and legumes.

6. Detoxify your emotions. It's the rare woman who can look radiant while feeling stressed, depressed, angry, or anxious. You owe it to yourself to address the problems in your life that are aging you prematurely. Sometimes only your subconscious is aware of these issues, but because there is an emotional aspect to detoxifying the body, feelings of grief, sadness, or resentment may surface during your detox. This is perfectly normal, and it gives you a chance to become aware of those feelings, and deal with them once and for all. If you experience "toxic emotions," be grateful they've come to the surface, acknowledge them, and then let them go. That way you can rid your body of any suppressed feelings, even if for no other reason than the fact that your liver will benefit.

How Your Liver Gives You Healthy Skin

Countless women have asked me the secret to beautiful skin at any age, desiring a clear, supple, wrinkle-free complexion. It's less of a mystery than you might think. Beautiful skin requires three things: Proper nutrition, a healthy lifestyle, and efficient detoxification pathways.

When you look in the mirror, your health is reflected in your skin. If you see blotchy, blemished, sagging, or sallow skin, it's likely that your body is having difficulty ridding itself of toxins and balancing your hormones. As I've said, this occurs when your liver, your body's main organ of detoxification, becomes overtaxed. Therefore, to improve your physical appearance, start by improving your liver's ability to cleanse your body of environmental toxins and natural waste.

For more on radiant beauty that starts on the inside, see Chapter Two.

Try these important and very helpful suggestions for creating the calm, peaceful, and positive emotions that are so necessary for healthy liver function and detoxification. Over the years, I've found these tips to be very helpful in neutralizing my own toxic emotions, as well as those of various family members and friends.

→ **Limit your exposure to toxic emotions in the environment.**
Two years ago I made the decision to shut off my television set and limit my consumption of the news. The media—whether it's television, radio, or newspaper—specializes in presenting the news with violent, fearful, and scary images and stories that contain very little that is inspiring and uplifting.

Too much of this toxic input from the environment can literally overwhelm your body's ability to process and detoxify these negative and disturbing images, and can, in turn, significantly undermine your health, energy, and well-being.

→ **Spend more time appreciating yourself.** Women are notoriously hard on themselves. We are constantly criticizing ourselves for not being good enough, smart enough, beautiful enough, or thin enough. My women friends are always jokingly offering to give each other transplants of their most disliked body parts—usually the breasts, behinds, and stomachs—when they feel too large. Send positive messages to your body that reinforce your sense of self worth and self love.

In fact, why not spend just a few minutes a day thanking and appreciating your body, including your liver, and the hard work that it does detoxifying every second of the day and night? Write these positive thank yous and appreciative thoughts to your body as affirmations in your journal, say them out loud in the privacy of your bedroom or office, or even visualize sending loving messages to your body each day. Over time, releasing more and more of your own toxic emotions and replacing them with kind and loving thoughts to yourself will help to diminish the load on your detox system. Then your body will begin to be filled with more light, radiance, and health.

→ **Plan to incorporate time for reflection, meditation, or a quiet hobby, like reading.** Stretching or yoga will help calm emotional upsets and help keep you from reabsorbing toxins in your tissues.

Dry Brush Massage

Also, to facilitate detoxification, I highly recommend giving yourself a dry brush massage. Dry brushing stimulates the lymphatic system, which helps move fluids through the body and carries toxins to the liver for detoxification and elimination.

To give yourself a dry-brush massage, use a moderately soft, natural vegetable-fiber bristle brush, and rub the skin vigorously to stimulate it and remove dead cells. Then, brush your body using short, brisk strokes. The following brush sequence will help move toxins from the periphery of the body towards your center, where the liver can eliminate them. Brush:

→ From your feet toward your pelvis
→ From your wrists to your armpits
→ From your chin to the navel

Brush gently at first, because your body is likely to be sensitive to this treatment. The massage should take about 10 minutes per day and should be continued for one to three months, at which time you can dry-brush twice per week as part of a preventive maintenance program. You can add sea salt to the brush if you want to open your pores further to intensify the cleansing effect of the massage.

Detoxifying Foods

Certain foods have been known to be liver-friendly since ancient times. Just so you are clear on why, I've compiled a list of the components in the foods that can help you perform that inner "spring cleaning"—any time of year:

- **Artichokes and broccoli** contain bitter constituents that strengthen glands that produce digestive juices, stimulate the gallbladder, and encourage fat digestion.

- **Broccoli** and **green cabbage** contain calcium, which combats lead and cadmium storage in the body.

- **Grains, leafy greens, peas, carrots, potatoes, apples, pears,** and **berries** contain fiber that stimulates the intestines and soaks up metabolic and other waste so that you can eliminate them.

- Spices such as **ginger, chiles, pepper,** and **paprika** contain heat that stimulates digestion.

- **Peas, beans, spinach, nuts, cabbage,** and **grapes** contain iron, which promotes blood formation and oxygen transport.

- **Cabbage, radishes, root veggies, onions,** and **leeks** contain mustard oils that purify and have an antiseptic effect, bolster stomach and intestine activity, and strengthen liver, gallbladder, kidneys, and bladder.

- **Potatoes, cabbage, brown rice, fruit,** and **grains** contain potassium, which rids your body of excess fluid, stimulates kidney function, and strengthens blood vessels and kidneys.

- **Fruit** and **vegetables** contain secondary plant substances that provide free-radical protection, help the cleansing process, and can be diuretic.

- Almost all **fruits and veggies, red cabbage, grains, and nuts** contain selenium, which binds heavy metals and enables their elimination from your body, stimulates the liver, and deactivates free radicals.

- **Fennel, carrots,** and **celery** contain volatile oils that stimulate metabolism, appetite, and digestion; cleanse mucous membranes; and strengthen the stomach, liver, gallbladder, and intestines.

- **Fish, meat,** and **grains** contain zinc, which helps combat stress and lessens the liver's burden.

Detox Recipes

Cleansing your body from the inside out is a great way to improve your skin's appearance, as well as to lose weight, restore your health, and improve your overall physical appearance. The following recipes, starring nutrient-blessed, liver-loving foods lead the way to a vibrant, super-vital you.

Shakes & Drinks

Apple, Mango, & Ginger Soother   Serves 2

Spices such as ginger, chiles, pepper, and paprika contain hot constituents that stimulate digestion. Ginger is also one of the most effective remedies for nausea and has been used as an aphrodisiac for centuries.

  2 large apples (e.g., Cox, Rome Beauty, or McIntosh)
  1 medium mango
  ¾-inch-piece fresh ginger

Wash and slice the apples, peel and chop the mango, and peel the ginger with a vegetable peeler.

Using a juicer, juice together the ingredients. Add ice cubes and enjoy.

BoysenNana Smoothie   Serves 2

This frothy beverage is high in estrogen-combating potassium and magnesium.

  1 frozen banana
  1 cup boysenberries
  ½ cup organic apple juice
  ½ cup almond milk
  ½ cup ground flax

Break frozen banana into chunks.

Place all ingredients in a blender. Blend until smooth, adding more juice or milk for thinner consistency.

Pear & Kiwi Smoothie   Serves 2

This luscious smoothie is a sweet way to start a morning. One kiwi packs in 95 percent of a day's vitamin C.

1 pear
1 banana
3 kiwi
¼ cup fresh pineapple
1 cup freshly juiced apple juice or organic, unfiltered from a bottle
4 ½ tablespoon soy yogurt
¼ cup ground flax

Core pear but do not peel. Peel banana and kiwis. Then place all ingredients into food processor and blend till frothy, adding more apple juice for thinner consistency, if desired.

Pour into two glasses and serve.

Tropical Tofu Smoothie   Serves 2

Isoflavone-rich soy foods, such as tofu, take the edge off of estrogen dominance by making it harder for your body's own, more potent estrogen to bind to the receptors.

⅔ cup soft tofu (3 ounces), drained
1 cup cubed pineapple, chilled
1 cup sliced mango, chilled
½ cup vanilla-flavored soy yogurt (fortified with calcium, if possible)
⅓ cup papaya nectar
1 teaspoon xylitol
Dash of ground nutmeg (optional)

Place tofu in a blender; process until smooth. Add pineapple and next four ingredients; process until smooth.

Serve immediately. Sprinkle with nutmeg, if desired.

Carrot & Mango Blend   Serves 2

In addition to being rich in vitamin A, carrots are high in alpha-carotene, an antioxidant 10 times more effective than beta-carotene in suppressing lung, liver, and skin cancer, and 38 percent stronger in antioxidant activity than beta-carotene.

    3 large carrots
    1 medium mango

Peel and trim the washed carrots. Peel and chop mango.

Using a juicer, juice together the ingredients. Add ice and enjoy.

Ginger-Turmeric Toddy   Serves 2

The medicinally active compound in turmeric is curcumin, which increases bile secretion and contraction of the gallbladder, thereby facilitating detoxification. It is a free-radical-fighting, antioxidant-rich curry spice; while tummy-soothing ginger was known in ancient times as the spice of "burning desire."

    2 ½ cups spring or filtered water
    2 teaspoons xylitol
    2 teaspoons green tea (loose leaves or loose tea from 2 green tea bags)
    6 mint leaves, crushed

Heat water to just below boiling point. Combine xylitol, green tea, and mint in a medium bowl; cover with heated water and steep 5 minutes. Strain tea mixture through a fine sieve into a bowl; discard solids.

Serve hot in tea glasses or mugs.

> Green tea contains polyphenols, which appear to enhance the activity of your body's antioxidant and detoxifying enzymes, including such key enzymes as glutathione peroxidase and glutathione S-transferase. Mint relaxes muscles and soothes your mood.

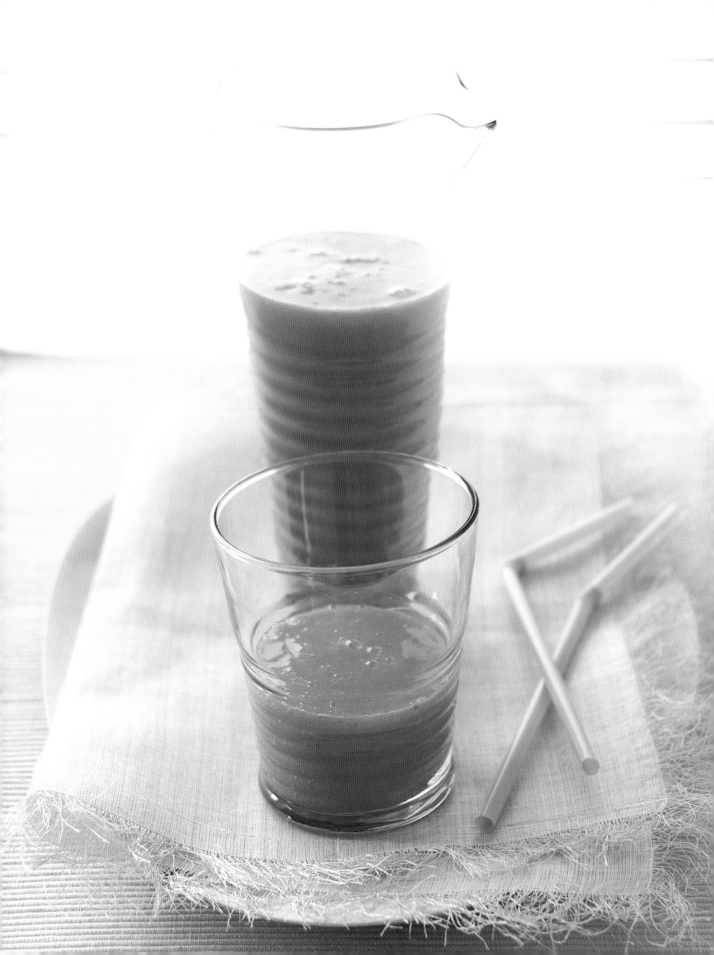

Snacks & Appetizers

Artichokes with Sorrel & Radish Dips Serves 2

Artichokes provide the vitamin-B complex, calcium, magnesium, and potassium vital to your health.

Salt to taste
Lemon slices
2 artichokes (about 18 ounces each)
1 egg
2 teaspoons Bragg Liquid Aminos
White pepper to taste
3–4 tablespoons olive oil
½ bunch fresh sorrel
¼ cup dairy-free sour cream
½ bunch radishes
2 ounces dairy-free cream cheese (e.g., Soya Kaas or Tofutti)
4–5 tablespoons rice milk
Ground cardamom to taste

After rinsing the artichokes, scissor off the thorny tops of the outside leaves and remove stems. In a large pot, heat a large amount of water with a few slices of lemon. Put the artichokes in the pot and boil over medium heat for 40 minutes, or when the leaves can be pulled away easily.

Boil the egg for 10 minutes, until the yolk is cooked hard. Peel and rinse the egg and separate the yolk from the white. Put the yolk through a fine sieve and mix it with the Bragg's, salt, and pepper.

Beat in the oil gradually. Wash the sorrel, shake dry, remove stalks, and chop the leaves. Mince the egg white and stir, with the sorrel and sour cream, into the yolk mixture. Season to taste; the mixture should be tangy.

Trim and grate the washed radishes. Stir together the cream cheese and rice milk, season with salt, pepper, and a little cardamom. Next stir in the radishes.

Drain the cooked artichokes and serve with the dips.

Baked Potato Chips Serves 4

Potatoes are a great source of both magnesium and potassium, stars in the legion of estrogen combatants.

20 ounces russet potatoes, with skin
1–2 teaspoons Bragg Liquid Aminos
1 pinch miso or seasoning blend (e.g., Mrs. Dash)
Freshly ground black pepper to taste

Place oven rack in center of oven. Preheat oven to 350°F.

Scrub and slice potatoes ⅛-inch thick, leaving their skin on. Arrange slices directly onto oven rack in a single layer; bake until golden brown and crispy, about 8–10 minutes.

Place in serving bowl and sprinkle with Bragg Liquid Aminos and seasonings.

Brown Rice Muffins Makes 12

Brown rice is one of the world's healthiest foods; its flour lends a nutty, soft texture to muffins.

2 cups brown rice flour
3 teaspoons baking powder
1–2 eggs
1 cup rice or nut milk
¼ cup canola oil
2 tablespoons xylitol

Combine the dry ingredients in a bowl. In a separate, small bowl, combine the eggs, milk, canola oil, and xylitol. Mix well and pour the batter into oiled muffin tins.

Bake at 400°F for about 15 minutes.

Bell Pepper Pineapple Salsa   Serves 2

Did you know peppers have a low pH and are high in both vitamin C and bioflavonoids, a powerful 1–2 punch that has been shown to help treat women with heavy periods?

    10 ounces pineapple
    ½ red bell pepper
    ½ small red onion
    1 tablespoon lime juice
    Salt to taste
    Tabasco sauce to taste
    2 teaspoons olive oil
    1 tablespoon chopped fresh cilantro
    Baked, organic corn tortilla chips

Cut off the pineapple rind from the sides, removing as much of the "eyes" as possible. Slice fruit lengthwise into quarters, and remove the core. Cut into small chunks. Dice the bell pepper. Peel and finely chop the onion. Stir together the pineapple, bell pepper, onion, lime juice, salt, Tabasco, olive oil, and cilantro.

Serve with tortilla chips.

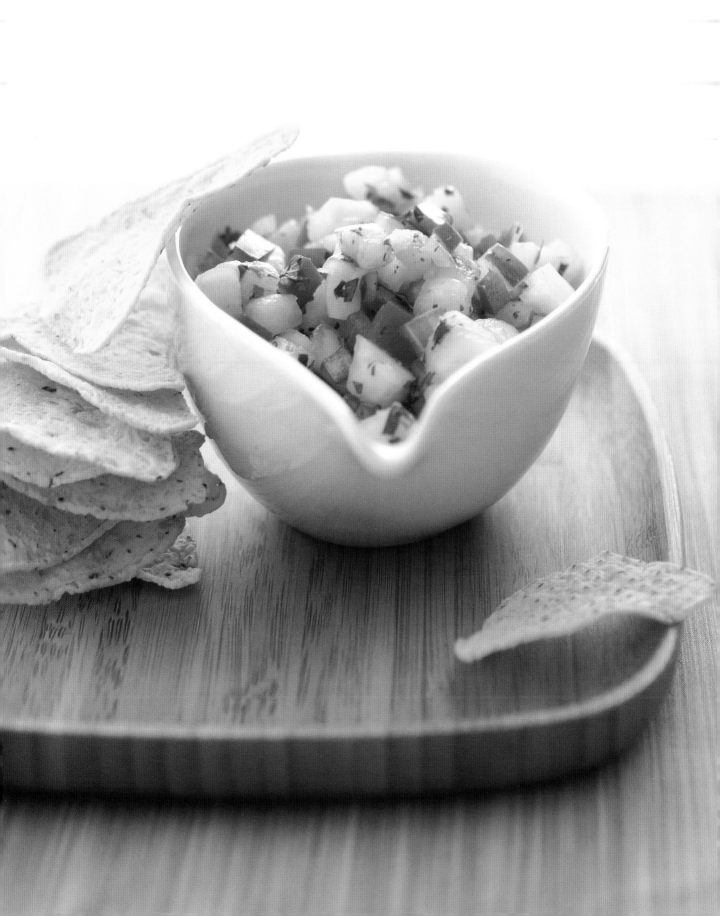

Cornmeal Johnnycakes with Radish Salad Serves 2

Also called hoecakes, johnnycakes date back to the 1700s. This version sidles up to nutrient-rich radish salad.

½ cup vegetable stock
⅓ cup finely ground cornmeal
1 small carrot
1 small kohlrabi
½ egg
½–1 bunch fresh dill
Salt to taste
Black pepper to taste
2–3 tablespoons cornmeal
3 tablespoons vegetable oil
¾ bunch radishes
2 tablespoons soy yogurt
1 tablespoon dairy-free cream cheese (e.g., Soya Kaas or Tofutti)
⅛ teaspoon ground cumin

In a medium pot, bring the vegetable stock to boil. Add the cornmeal and cook over low heat, tightly covered, for 10 minutes. Peel the carrot and kohlrabi and grate finely. Add the vegetables to the cornmeal and cook together for another 5 minutes. Transfer to a bowl. Stir in the egg and let the mixture cool for a while.

Wash the dill and remove feathery leaves from stalks. Stir the dill into the cornmeal mixture and season with salt and pepper. Add enough cornmeal to create a dough that binds well. Divide the dough and shape into 4 equal-sized patties. Heat the oil in a non-stick skillet over medium-high heat. Fry the johnnycake patties in the oil for 10 minutes over very low heat, turning cakes occasionally.

Meanwhile, wash the radishes and coarsely grate them. Stir together the grated radishes, soy yogurt, and cream cheese. Season with salt, pepper, and cumin. Serve atop or beside the johnnycakes.

GORP Deluxe Makes 2 cups

GORP stands for good ol' raisins and peanuts—standard trail mix fare. This nutritious and not-so-standard version can hit the ground running and satisfy homebodies, too. Plus, it's easy to substitute in a variety of your favorite nuts, seeds, and dried fruits.

¼ cup raisins
¼ cup unsalted peanuts or almonds
¼ cup soy nuts
¼ cup toasted sunflower seeds
¼ cup lightly salted pumpkin seeds
¼ cup dried cherries
¼ cup dried, unsulfured mangoes, cut into bite-sized pieces
¼ cup carob chips

In a bowl, combine the ingredients.

Place in sealed containers for the trail or store in the refrigerator for snacking.

Tangy Artichoke Dip Makes about 2 cups

This dip is a luscious accompaniment to fresh vegetables of any shape, size, or color.

2 green onions
1 cup canned artichokes packed in water, drained
½ teaspoon onion powder
1 cup dairy-free sour cream
2–3 tablespoons rice or nut milk

Wash and dice the green onions, then put them into food processor or blender with other ingredients, and blend until smooth.

Chill before serving.

Veggie Skewers Serves 4

Try serving these skewers with the Tangy Artichoke Dip on page 163.

1 package button mushrooms
1 small head broccoli
1 celery stalk
1 small zucchini
1 medium green or red bell pepper
8 bamboo skewers (9-inches long)

Rinse and dry the mushrooms. Wash and cut broccoli into 1-inch florets. Wash and cut remaining vegetables into 1-inch pieces. On each skewer, spear 1 mushroom, and 1 piece of celery, broccoli, zucchini, and bell pepper.

Serve with dip.

Breakfast

Baked Oatmeal Serves 6

Scientifically known as Avena sativa, oats lower cholesterol, reduce risk of cardiovascular disease, enhance immune response, and contain powerful phytonutrients whose anti-cancer activity is equal to or higher than that of fruits and veggies.

 3 cups oatmeal
 ½ cup xylitol
 2 teaspoons baking powder
 ½ teaspoon cinnamon
 ½ teaspoon salt
 ½ cup plain applesauce
 1 teaspoon vanilla
 2 eggs
 1 cup rice milk
 ½–1 cup raisins or blueberries
 Canola oil spray
 Honey to taste

Preheat oven to 350°F.

Mix the dry ingredients in 1 bowl. Mix the wet ingredients in another bowl. Stir the wet and dry ingredients together and add the raisins or blueberries.

Spread in a 9-inch x 9-inch pan, lightly sprayed with canola oil. Bake 20–30 minutes.

Serve plain or try it drizzled with honey, nut milk, or soy yogurt over the top.

Asparagus and Herb Omelet Serves 2

This is quick to make and features cleansing asparagus, which contains aspartic acid and potassium to stimulate the kidneys and help your body expel excess liquid.

    9 ounces green asparagus
    Salt to taste
    2 tablespoons canola oil
    1 teaspoon honey
    4 eggs
    2 tablespoons rice or nut milk
    White pepper to taste
    2 tablespoons chopped fresh Italian parsley
    1–2 tablespoons chopped fresh cilantro
    1–2 tablespoons chopped fresh chervil

Wash, trim and peel the asparagus. Steam it for 5–8 minutes over boiling, salted water, adding 1 teaspoon of the oil and the honey.

Whisk together the eggs, milk, salt, pepper, and herbs in a bowl.

Make one omelet at a time in a nonstick skillet with the remaining oil.

Drain the asparagus well, divide into two portions, wrap in the two omelets, and serve.

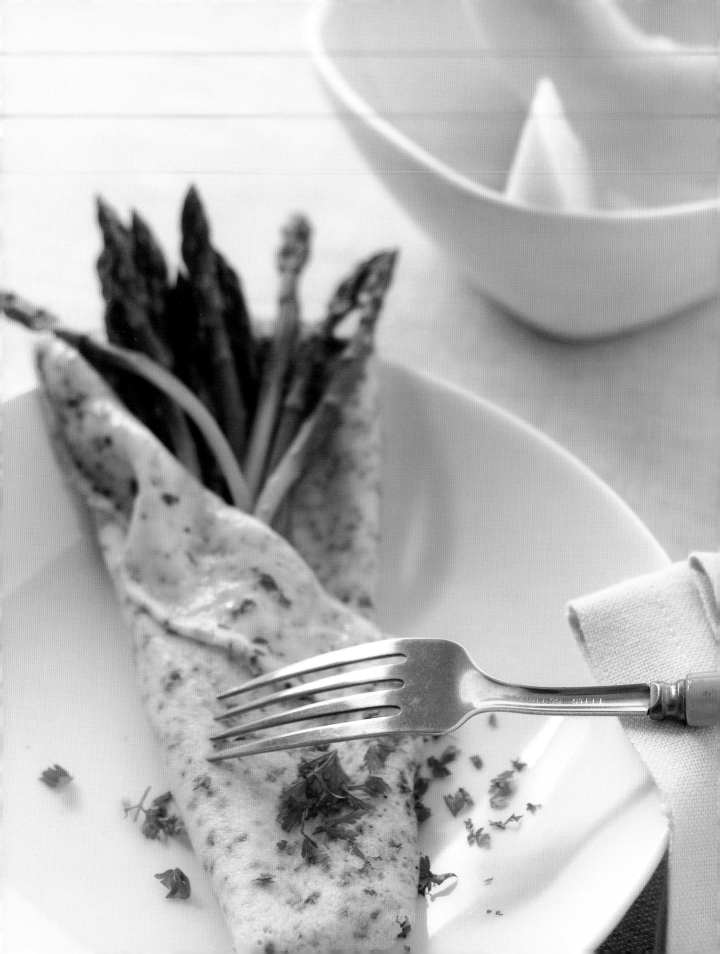

Blackberry Fool Serves 2

A fool is an old-fashioned English dessert traditionally made from cooked fruit folded into whipped cream. This fresh-fruit version makes a healthy breakfast or dessert.

    6 ounces fresh blackberries
    6 ounces soy yoghurt
    1 ½ tablespoons clear honey

Put the ingredients in a small bowl and whisk vigorously with a fork so that the raspberries break up, coloring the creamy mixture. Continue mixing until you have an even consistency.

Serve immediately.

Caffeine

If you habitually drink too much coffee or cola, or indulge in a chocolate bar every afternoon, you're putting undue stress on your adrenal glands, which secrete stress hormones. The caffeine stimulates the release of additional stress hormones, increasing your nervousness and anxiety and stealing valuable nutrients from the rest of your body to feed your overcharged, stressed nervous system. Caffeine can also affect estrogen levels, increasing blood levels of this hormone and thus contributing to menstrual problems as well as certain cancers.

Overall, caffeine also:
→ Triggers anxiety and panic symptoms;
→ Acts as a diuretic, speeding elimination of many valuable minerals and vitamins you need;
→ Increases frequency of hot flashes;
→ Reduces absorption of iron and calcium;
→ Worsens breast pain;
→ Raises blood levels of cholesterol and triglycerides, increasing your risk of heart disease; and
→ Increases acid production in the stomach, a risk factor for numerous gastrointestinal upsets

Brown Rice & Celery Root Griddlecakes with Herbed Yogurt Serves 2

Celery root, also known as celeriac, has diuretic properties, stimulates the appetite, aids digestion, and supports the lymphatic, nervous, and urinary systems.

½ cup brown rice
5 tablespoons soy yogurt
1 tablespoon dairy-free cream cheese (e.g., Soya Kaas or Tofutti)
Salt to taste
White pepper to taste
2 tablespoons chopped fresh herbs
1 tablespoon ground flaxseed
1 teaspoon unfiltered apple juice
5 ounces celery root
2 eggs

Cook rice in 1 cup water until tender but still firm, about 30 minutes. Stir together the soy yogurt, cream cheese, salt, pepper, herbs, flaxseed, and apple juice.

Peel and coarsely chop the celery root. Drain and cool the rice, and mix it with the root and eggs. Season with salt and pepper.

Over medium-high heat, heat a small portion of oil in a large skillet. Drop spoonfuls of the rice batter into the skillet to fry. Serve the small griddlecakes with the herbed yogurt.

Fruit Eye-Opener Serves 2

This sweet mix of carbohydrates and proteins will boost your energy while keeping the hunger pangs at bay.

- 1 apple or pear, cored and cubed
- 1 cup berries of varying hues
- 1 tablespoon xylitol
- 1 cup soy yogurt
- ½ cup organic granola

In individual serving bowls or parfait glasses, place the mixed fruit, in layers if you like.

Stir xylitol into the yogurt and pour about ½ cup of the yogurt mixture over the top of the fruit in each bowl.

Sprinkle with granola.

Oat Porridge Serves 1

Unrefined grains, such as oats, provide fiber, protein, carbohydrates, fats, B complex and other important vitamins, as well as a wealth of minerals, including calcium, magnesium, potassium, iron, copper, and manganese.

- ½ cup rice milk
- 3 tablespoons rolled oats (not instant)
- 1 tablespoon raisins
- 1 tablespoon raspberries
- 1 teaspoon honey

Heat the milk in a pan until almost boiling. Add the rolled oats and stir for about 2 ½–3 minutes. Pour into a bowl to serve.

Serve as a basic hot cereal or add all or any combination of the raisins, berries, and honey as a tasty topping.

Stewed Apricots Serves 3

Dried apricots are chock full of magnesium and potassium, key detoxifying agents.

  1 cup dried coarsely chopped apricots
  ¼ teaspoon cinnamon
  1 tablespoon honey or to taste
  1 cup water

Put apricots, cinnamon, and honey in medium saucepan and cover with water. Bring to boil over medium heat, then gently simmer over low heat for 20–30 minutes until apricots are tender.

Serve over Warm Wake-Up Cereal (see below) for a healthy start to any morning.

Warm Wake-Up Cereal Serves 3

This warm bowl of whole grains, seeds, and nuts perfectly complements the Stewed Apricots above.

  1 cup whole multigrain, wheat-free cereal or old-fashioned rolled oats (not instant)
  2–3 cups water (as directed on package)
  ½ cup mixed pumpkin seeds, sunflower seeds, and toasted, slivered almonds

Boil water over medium-high heat. Stir in oats or multigrains, cover, lower heat, and simmer until done (as directed).

Stir in seeds and nuts when cereal is cooked.

Lunch

Asparagus & Greens Sauté Serves 2

High in potassium and low in sodium, asparagus contains a special carbohydrate called inulin, which boosts growth and activity of friendly flora in your intestinal tract.

1 cucumber
9 ounces asparagus
1 bunch fresh arugula
9 ounces fresh spinach
1 onion
1 clove garlic
1 tablespoon olive oil
Sea salt to taste
Black pepper to taste
Ground nutmeg to taste
2 teaspoons borage oil
2 ounces soy Parmesan cheese

Wash the cucumber and halve it lengthwise. Seed it and cut it into ½-inch slices. Wash and trim the asparagus. Peel the bottom third of the spears, and cut into ¾–1-inch bites. Wash the arugula and spinach, shake dry, and finely chop. Skin and dice the onion and garlic.

In a skillet, heat the olive oil over medium heat. Add the onion and garlic and sauté until translucent. Add the asparagus and the cucumber. Season with salt, pepper, nutmeg, and cover tightly. Simmer lightly for about 10 minutes over low. Add the arugula and spinach, season with salt and pepper, and simmer for another 3 minutes.

Serve the vegetables on plates, sprinkle with borage oil, and grate the soy Parmesan on top.

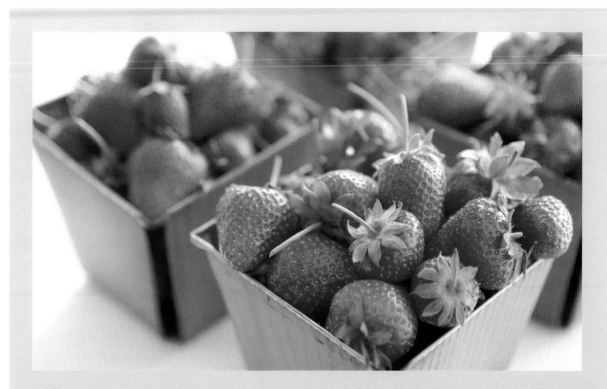

Plant Foods with Magnesium and Potassium A-plenty

Your body and mind need constant nourishing and rejuvenation to deal with everyday stress in our fast-paced world. Eating food high in magnesium and potassium can help to boost your energy naturally and unleash a steady stream of vigor that lasts all day. I recommend three to five servings of fresh fruit and three servings of vegetables each day. I also encourage adding whole grains and legumes to your diet according to your personal tolerances and needs. For example, if you need to eat meat several times a week to feel your best, don't leave out grains and legumes; but if you eat vegetarian meals some or all of the time, try to work grains and legumes into your diet. If your goal is to maintain already good energy levels, be sure that at least a few of those daily fruit and vegetable choices come from the lists of potassium- and magnesium-rich foods on this page. If your energy levels are low, select the majority of your fruits and vegetables from these lists. Be sure to get your share of oil-rich seeds and nuts. If your tolerances permit, add four servings of legumes each week and liberal amounts of whole grains.

Great plant sources of both magnesium and potassium:

Vegetables and legumes: globe artichoke, asparagus, black eyed peas, beets, broccoli, collard greens, sweet corn, kale, lima beans, okra, parsnips, green peas, potato (especially with skin on), pumpkin, sauerkraut, spinach, squash (especially winter varieties), sweet potato, tomato, tomato paste, turnips, vegetable juice cocktail, yams.

Fruits: dried apricots, avocado, banana, blackberries, black currants, dates, dried figs, kiwi fruit, cantaloupe, orange, papaya, dried peach, dried pear, dried prunes, raisins, strawberries.

Grains: barley, cornmeal, millet, brown rice, wild rice.

Cabbage and Apple Slaw Serves 2

The beneficial phytochemicals in cabbage help trigger and stabilize your body's antioxidant and detoxification systems.

2 sweet apples (e.g., galas or Braeburns)
7 ounces cabbage (from a pre-shredded, bagged coleslaw mix)
½ cup sauerkraut juice
2–3 tablespoons Bragg Liquid Aminos
Sea salt to taste
Black pepper to taste
¾ cup dairy-free sour cream
½ bunch fresh dill
¼ cup coarsely chopped walnuts
½ teaspoon anise seeds
½ teaspoon poppy seeds
½ teaspoon flaxseeds
1 tablespoon canola oil

Wash, dry, and grate the apples, leaving their peel on. In a bowl, combine the shredded cabbage and grated apple. Stir the sauerkraut juice and Bragg's into the apple and cabbage mix. Season with salt and pepper.

Let the slaw stand for about 1 hour to meld the flavors. Meanwhile, wash and shake dry the dill and chop the leaves.

To make the dressing, stir together the sour cream, chopped dill, walnuts, anise and poppy seeds, flaxseeds, and canola oil. Stir the dressing into the slaw, seasoning again with salt and pepper to taste.

Chinese Chicken Soup Serves 4

Chicken's mix of B-complex vitamins makes it a helpful food in supporting energy metabolism throughout the body, while ginger relaxes and soothes the intestinal tract and possesses antioxidant effects.

1 tablespoon canola oil
1 cup chopped onion
1 tablespoon diced, peeled fresh ginger
3 garlic cloves, minced
½ pound skinless, boneless chicken breast, cut into 1-inch pieces
1 ½ cups water
2 ¾ cups reduced-sodium chicken broth
1 ½ cups corn
2 bags ginseng tea (or 1 sliced ginseng root)
⅛ teaspoon white miso
Dash of white pepper

Heat the oil in a Dutch oven over medium-high heat. Add onion, ginger, and garlic cloves; sauté 2 minutes. Add chicken; sauté 4 minutes. Add water and broth; bring to a boil. Stir in corn and ginseng tea; bring to a boil. Reduce heat; simmer 20 minutes.

Season with miso and pepper.

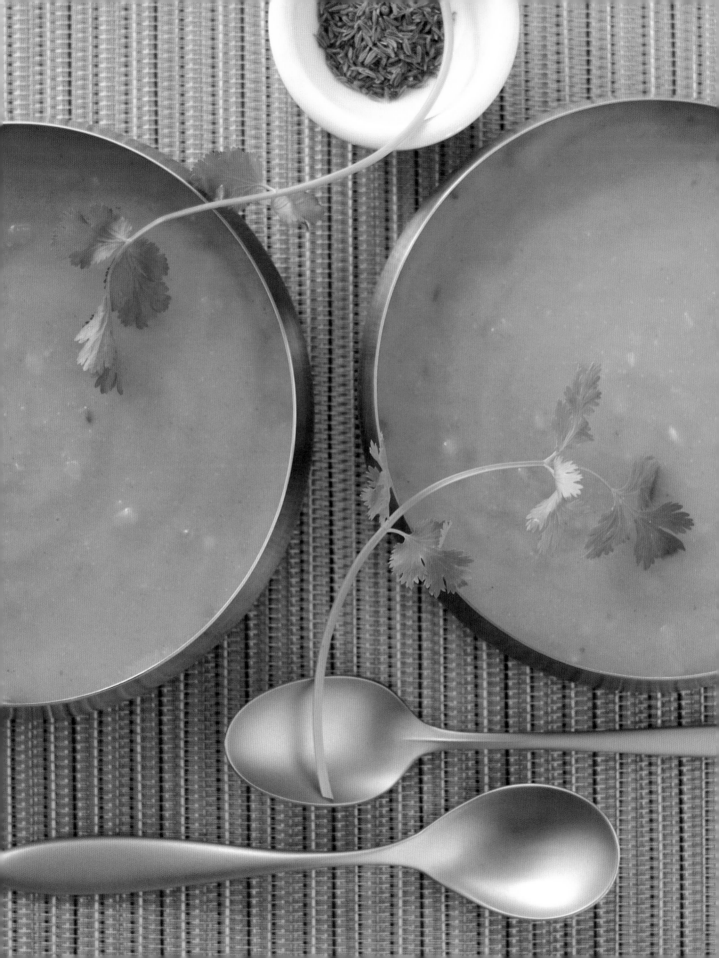

East Indian Lentil Soup Serves 4

Fiber-rich lentils increase your energy by replenishing your iron stores, while the active compound in turmeric—curcumin—facilitates detoxification.

2 ⅓ cups water
1 ½ cups red lentils
1 teaspoon xylitol
¼ teaspoon ground turmeric
1 can vegetable broth (14.5-ounce)
½ teaspoon cumin seeds
1 tablespoon olive oil
1 ½ cups minced onion
3 garlic cloves, minced
1 tablespoon fresh lime juice
⅛ teaspoon miso
⅛ teaspoon crushed red pepper flakes
Cilantro sprigs

In a medium saucepan, combine 1 ⅓ water, red lentils, xylitol, turmeric, and broth. Bring to a boil, cover, reduce heat, and simmer 10 minutes or until lentils are very tender. Cool slightly. Carefully pour lentil mixture into a food processor or blender; process until smooth. Set aside.

In a large nonstick skillet over medium heat, toast the cumin seeds in olive oil for 30 seconds or until fragrant and lightly browned. Peel and mince onion and garlic. Add to skillet and sauté 10 minutes or until lightly browned. Stir in puréed lentil mixture, remaining 1 cup water, lime juice, miso, and red pepper flakes; cook until thoroughly heated.

Ladle into bowls and garnish with cilantro.

Lux Lox Soup Serves 2

Choose wild, rather than farm-raised, smoked salmon. Studies show that wild salmon have lower levels of toxins than their farmed brethren.

10 ounces white or green asparagus
2 cups water
Salt to taste
Honey to taste
2 tablespoons canola oil
4 ounces fresh peas in the pod (about 2 ounces when shelled; or 2 ounces frozen peas, thawed)
4 ounces smoked salmon
1 tablespoon fresh lemon juice, including pulp
1 tablespoon rice flour
⅛ cup dairy-free sour cream
⅛ cup rice milk

Rinse the asparagus, snap off the tough ends, peel the bottom third of the spears, and reserve the trimmings and peelings. Snip off the tips and set aside, covered. Roughly chop the asparagus spears and put in a saucepan with 1 cup water, a pinch of salt, a dash of honey, and ½ teaspoon of canola oil. Bring to a boil, cover, and cook for 15 minutes. Purée the cooked asparagus pieces with their cooking liquid.

Meanwhile, put the asparagus trimmings and peelings into another saucepan. Add the remaining 1 cup water, a pinch of salt, dash of honey, and ½ teaspoon canola oil. Cover and simmer for 15 minutes. Strain and reserve the cooking liquid, throwing away the solids.

Next, shell the peas. Dice the salmon and sprinkle it with lemon juice.

Put the remaining oil in a saucepan over medium-low heat. Stir in the flour and cook until golden brown. Pour in the strained asparagus cooking liquid and mix well; add the asparagus purée, sour cream, and rice milk. Stir.

Mix the asparagus tips, peas, and salmon into the soup, and cook 2–3 minutes. Stir, season, and serve.

Quinoa Salad Serves 4

Quinoa is my favorite wheat substitute. This gluten-free seed from a leafy plant related to spinach is an excellent source of protein. It also contains high levels of potassium and vitamin B2, as well as vitamin B1, B3, B6, copper, magnesium, and zinc.

2 cups cooked rice, quinoa, or corn pasta
1 cup garbanzo beans
2/3 cup steamed chopped broccoli
1/4 cup diced red onion
1/4 cup diced green bell pepper
1/2 teaspoon basil
1/2 teaspoon tarragon
3 tablespoons olive oil
Juice of 1/2 lemon
1/8 teaspoon sea salt

Combine all ingredients in a large bowl. Mix well, then chill for at least 1 hour before serving.

Soup Marguerite Serves 2

This lycopene-rich recipe is inspired by Pizza Marguerite, which you can further simulate by dipping a piece of cornmeal bread into the bowl.

8 large fresh tomatoes
1 cup water
1/4 cup plus 1 teaspoon chopped fresh basil
Black pepper
2 teaspoons grated soy mozzarella

Halve the tomatoes, then roast them skin side up under a broiler until blackened. Put the tomatoes in a food processor, carefully adding 1 cup boiling water, 1/4 cup chopped basil, and a little black pepper. Blend until smooth, ladle into soup bowls, sprinkle soy mozzarella and remaining teaspoon basil over top, and serve.

Wild Rice Melange with Raspberry Vinaigrette Serves 2

You can make larger quantities of the raspberry vinaigrette to store in the refrigerator for a week. Toss with other veggies to make an insta-salad.

½ cup bean sprouts
½ cup chopped celery rib
¼ cup chopped walnuts
½ cup cooked wild rice
3 tablespoons sesame seeds
½ cup cooked red kidney beans (or from a can, rinsed and drained)
½ cup cubed ripe avocado

Vinaigrette

10 raspberries
1 tablespoon raspberry vinegar
1 tablespoon olive oil
1 teaspoon tamari

Halve the bean sprouts and dice the celery and walnuts, then add all ingredients, and place into a salad bowl.

Put the vinaigrette ingredients into a blender or food processor and blend for a few seconds. Pour it over the salad and toss to coat.

This dressing is great to make in a larger quantity and then store in an air-tight container in the fridge for a week or so.

Dinner

Chicken and Papaya Kebabs Serves 4

Chicken's B vitamins are involved as co-factors that help enzymes throughout the body guide metabolic reactions, while fibrous papayas are rich sources of antioxidant nutrients; potassium and magnesium; and the B vitamins, folic acid, and pantothenic acid.

2 tablespoons extra virgin olive oil
2 garlic cloves, crushed
½ teaspoon ground cumin
½ teaspoon ground turmeric
½ teaspoon paprika
2 teaspoons lemon juice
1 pound skinned boned chicken breasts, cut into 1-inch pieces
1 papaya, peeled and cut into 1-inch pieces
4 skewers (10-inches long)
Olive oil spray
Black beans
Brown rice

Combine first 7 ingredients in a bowl; stir well. Cover and marinate in refrigerator for 1–8 hours. Remove chicken from bowl, reserving marinade.

Thread chicken and papaya alternately onto skewers. Prepare grill or broiler. Place kebabs on grill rack or broiler pan coated with cooking spray; cook 7 minutes on each side or until done, basting occasionally with reserved marinade.

Cook black beans and brown rice according to package directions and serve with the kebabs.

Fish in Dill Sour Cream Serves 2

Anti-inflammatory nutrients in fish may help prevent or lessen the progression of asthma, rheumatoid arthritis, and migraine headaches. Nutrients in fish, such as cod and halibut, also promote detoxification and protect against ovarian and digestive tract cancers.

10–12 ounces fish fillets (e.g., cod, haddock, turbot, halibut, or monkfish)
Olive oil
1 teaspoon fresh lemon juice
1 tablespoon Bragg Liquid Aminos
2 teaspoons chopped fresh dill (or 3/4 teaspoon dried dill)
Sea salt and black pepper to taste
2–3 thick slices red onion
½ cup dairy-free sour cream

Preheat the oven to 375°F.

Rinse and pat dry the fish fillets and place them, skin side down, in an oiled baking pan. Sprinkle with lemon juice, Bragg's, dill, salt, and pepper. Break the red onion slices into rings and layer them in equal portions on each fillet. Spoon sour cream over the onion rings and the fillets, spreading evenly.

Cover pan and bake for 25–30 minutes, until fish is opaque and flakes easily with a fork.

Mashed Potatoes With Herring, Radishes & Chives   Serves 2

Brimming with health-promoting essential fatty acids, herring is good for skin radiance and provides cardiovascular benefits, while potatoes are magnesium- and potassium-rich.

14 ounces baking potatoes
Sea salt to taste
1 bunch fresh chives
1 bunch radishes
½ cup rice or soy milk
1 tablespoon canola oil
White pepper to taste
4 marinated or pickled herring fillets

Place potatoes in a pot with enough cold, salted water to cover. Bring to a boil, reduce the heat, and simmer until potatoes are tender, about 20–30 minutes. Drain potatoes and set aside.

Meanwhile, wash, shake dry, and finely chop the chives. Wash the radishes, setting aside four, plus a few leaves, for garnish. Dice the remaining radishes.

In a saucepan, simmer the potatoes with the milk and canola oil over medium heat. Mash the potatoes coarsely with a masher or fork. Stir in the chives and diced radishes, season with salt and pepper, and heat through.

Arrange herring fillets on plates with the mashed potatoes and reserved radishes. Chop the reserved radish leaves, sprinkle on the potatoes, and serve.

Lemon Shrimp with Three-Bean Salad Serves 2

Black-eyed peas are an excellent source of calcium and vitamin A; kidney beans are high in iron, and magnesium; and garbanzos, in vitamins B6, C, and zinc. All are fiber- and folate-rich.

½ red bell pepper
½ yellow bell pepper
4 ounces garbanzo beans (canned), drained
7 ounces black eyed peas (canned), drained
4 ounces red kidney beans (canned), drained
¼ cup finely chopped cilantro
4 teaspoons liquid honey
¼ cup Bragg Liquid Aminos
⅔ teaspoon paprika
6 ounces jumbo shrimp
1 ½ tablespoons minced parsley
2 tablespoons olive oil
1 tablespoon fresh lemon juice

Halve the bell peppers. Remove the stem, ribs and seeds, and rinse and thinly slice.

To make the salad, combine beans and bell peppers, add the cilantro, and toss.

In a bowl, whisk the honey, Bragg's, and paprika to an even consistency. Pour the dressing over the bean salad and toss thoroughly.

Peel, devein, and wash the shrimp. Sauté the shrimp in the olive oil in a wok or large skillet, stirring occasionally. Cook until pink on all sides and set aside.

Wash, shake dry, and mince the parsley. Sprinkle cooked shrimp with the lemon juice and parsley. On two dinner-sized plates, place bean salad and spoon shrimp over the top and serve.

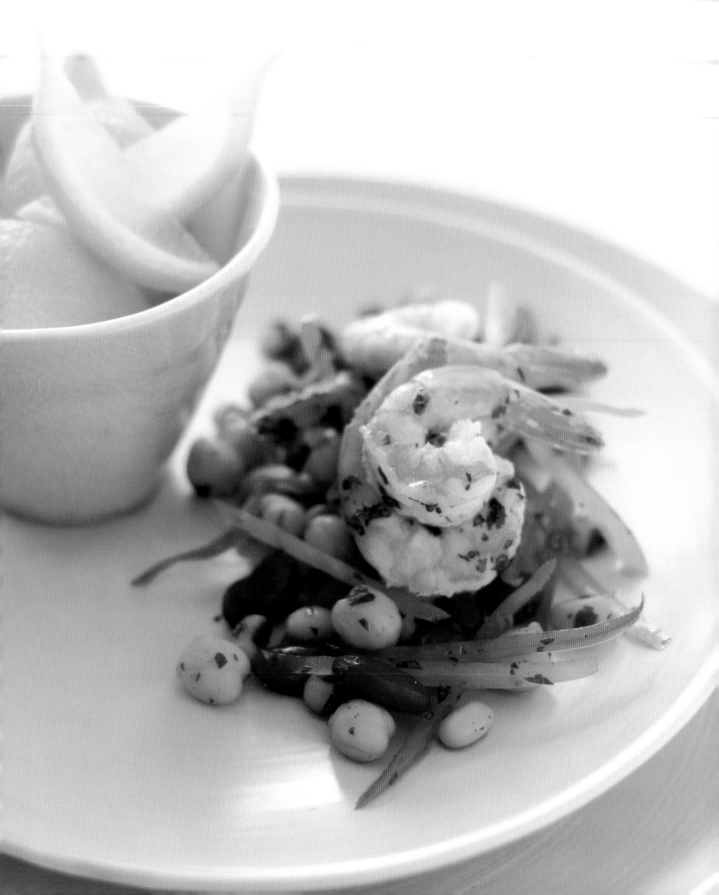

Pineapple Cashew Stew   Serves 4

Cashews are a good source of copper, which plays a role in your body's iron utilization, elimination of free radicals, development of bone and connective tissue, and your production of the skin and hair pigment called melanin.

    1 cup chopped onions
    1 teaspoon minced garlic
    1 tablespoon peanut oil
    1 bunch kale (about 4 cups sliced)
    2 cups crushed pineapple (20-ounce can), undrained
    ½ cup cashew butter
    Dash Tabasco
    ½ cup chopped fresh cilantro
    Sea salt to taste
    Cashews, crushed
    Green onions, chopped (optional)

In a saucepan, cover and cook the onions and garlic in peanut oil for about 10 minutes, stirring frequently, until onions are lightly browned.

Meanwhile, wash and shake dry the kale; greens from stems and discard stems and any yellowing leaves. Stack the greens, roll them, and slice into 1-inch ribbons.

Simmer the pineapple and its juice with the onions. Stir in the kale, cover, and simmer for about 5 minutes, stirring occasionally, until just tender. Mix in the cashew butter, Tabasco, and cilantro and simmer another 5 minutes.

Season with sea salt and top with cashews and/or green onions, if desired.

Portobello Quiche Serves 6

Portobellos are the fully mature form of cremini mushrooms, which maintain immune function, stem fatigue, and protect against breast cancer by preventing excessive estrogen buildup.

Olive oil
¾ cup diced red onion
3 portobello mushrooms, coarsely diced
2 cups chopped fresh spinach
¼ cup ground cornmeal
2 cups unflavored rice milk
4 eggs
¼ cup soy Parmesan cheese
1 ½ teaspoons garlic powder
1 ½ teaspoons Spike or other mixed spice seasoning
1 teaspoon pepper

Heat olive oil in skillet on medium high for several minutes. Add onion and portobellos and sauté for 4–5 minutes. Add spinach and cook 3–4 additional minutes. Mix in cornmeal thoroughly.

Place in a deep-dish pan—preferably a quiche pan or comparable dish—and set aside.

In a separate mixing bowl, whisk rice milk with the eggs and Parmesan. Add spices, then pour over the portobello mixture.

Bake at 350°F for 40–45 minutes, until the center is set and firm. Let stand 5–10 minutes before serving.

Tofu Burritos   Serves 4–6

In traditional Chinese medicine, tofu is among those foods known for their ability to cleanse and restore liver function.

3 garlic cloves
1 red bell pepper
2 medium onions (about 2 cups), finely chopped
2 cakes firm tofu
3 tablespoons vegetable oil
¼ teaspoon cayenne
2 teaspoons paprika
1 tablespoon ground cumin
1 teaspoon ground coriander
1 teaspoon dried oregano
½ cup corn
¼ cup tomato paste
2 tablespoons Bragg Liquid Aminos
Salt and black pepper to taste
6 spelt flour tortillas (10-inches each)
Salsa (optional)

Peel and press or mince the garlic cloves; rinse and dice the bell pepper and finely chop the onions. Crumble the tofu.

Heat oil in a large skillet over medium heat, sauté the garlic, cayenne, and onions for 1–2 minutes. Add the bell peppers, continuing to sauté. When the onions are softened and opaque, add the paprika, cumin, coriander, oregano, corn, and tofu; continue to sauté.

Preheat oven to 350°F.

When the vegetables are tender, stir in the tomato paste and Bragg's; season with salt and pepper to taste.

Into the middle of each tortilla, spoon about ¾ cup veggie filling and roll it up burrito-style. Place the burritos side-by-side in a lightly oiled baking dish, covered tightly with aluminum foil. Bake 20 minutes.

Serve warm, topped with Bell Pepper Pineapple Salsa (see page 160), if you want to add a bit of spicy flavor to your burrito.

Turkey in Coconut Milk with Wild Rice   Serves 2

Research has shown that natural, unprocessed coconut fat in the diet leads to a normalization of body lipids, protects against alcohol damage to the liver, and improves the immune system's anti-inflammatory response.

¾ cup wild rice
2 cups water
Sea salt to taste
10 ounces boneless turkey breast
White pepper to taste
8 ounces asparagus
½ fresh pineapple (about 9 ounces)
1 tablespoon vegetable oil
1 ⅔ cups unsweetened coconut milk
1 teaspoon sambal bajak (Asian markets) or allspice
3 teaspoons arrowroot
Wild rice

Rinse wild rice. Combine in a large saucepan rice, water, and salt. Bring to a boil. Stir once, cover, and simmer over low heat until the water is absorbed and the rice is fluffy and tender, about 35–50 minutes.

Meanwhile, season the turkey with salt and pepper and cut into thin strips. Peel the lower third of the asparagus stalks, then diagonally slice them into 1-inch pieces. Peel, core, and cube the pineapple.

Heat the oil in a skillet. Brown the turkey strips over medium heat. Add the asparagus and cook for 3–5 minutes, stirring constantly. Stir in the coconut milk and sambal bajak and simmer over low heat for another 6 minutes. Dissolve the arrowroot in a little water and stir it into the skillet. Finally, add the pineapple and cook until heated through.

Cook wild rice according to package directions and serve with this dish.

Desserts

Basque Fruit Compote   Serves 8

This dessert, which hails from the Basque country, uses both fresh and dried fruit. Serve it alone or spooned over dairy-free yogurt, rice-flour pound cake, or brown rice.

    6 dried figs
    6 prunes
    6 dried apricots
    ½ cup golden raisins
    ½ cup freshly juiced apple or unfiltered, organic bottled apple juice
    1 cup freshly juiced or food-processed red grapes, skins left on
    1 cup water
    ¼ cup honey
    1 teaspoon grated lemon rind
    2 teaspoons grated orange rind
    1 apple, peeled and cut into 12 wedges
    1 pear, peeled and cut into 12 wedges

Microwave the first five ingredients in a microwave-safe bowl on high for 1 minute. Set aside.

In a medium saucepan, vigorously stir together grape juice, water, honey, and rinds. Bring to a boil. Add dry fruit mixture, cover, reduce heat, and simmer 10 minutes, stirring occasionally. Add apple, cover, and cook 5 minutes, stirring occasionally. Add pear, cover, and cook 5 minutes, intermittently stirring.

Remove from heat. Cover and let stand at room temperature 2 hours before serving.

Berries with Yogurt Cream Serves 2

From antioxidants that fight cancer and heart disease to bioflavonoids and minerals essential for energy and good bones, the nutrients in berries benefit your whole body.

    4 ounces soy yogurt
    1 ½ tablespoons honey, or more to taste
    2 tablespoons rice milk
    ½ teaspoon ground cinnamon, plus more for garnish
    ½ lemon
    2 ounces small fresh raspberries
    2 ounces fresh blackberries
    2 ounces fresh blueberries
    2 ounces small seedless grapes or red currants
    2 fresh plums

Combine the soy yogurt with ½ tablespoon honey, rice milk, and a pinch of the ground cinnamon; and divide among two dessert plates.

Thoroughly rinse and dry the lemon. Finely grate the zest and squeeze the juice. Mix the zest and juice in a bowl with remaining 1 tablespoon honey (or more to taste).

Wash and drain the berries and grapes or currants. Wash and stone the plums, and cut into segments. Gently stir the plums segments into the lemon juice mixture.

Arrange all fruit on top of the yogurt, sprinkle with cinnamon, and serve.

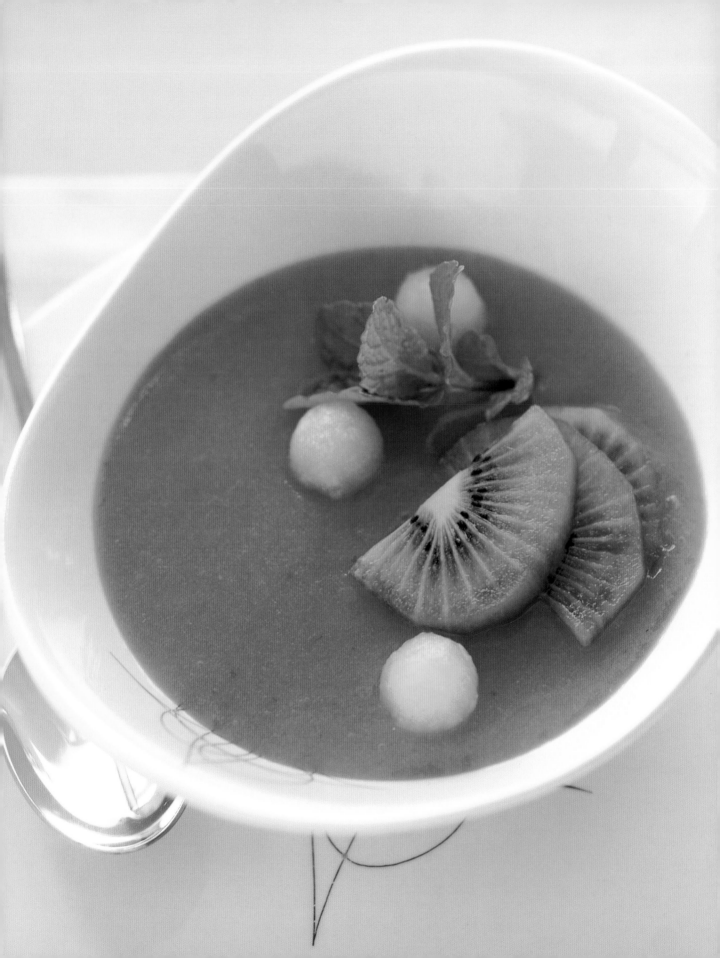

MeloMango & KiwiBerry Soup Serves 2

Melons, mangoes, and kiwis are super-low in calories, while super-high in vitamins and cleansing nutrients.

⅔ cup strawberries, well chilled
½ ripe melon (e.g., cantaloupe), well chilled
1 small, ripe mango, well chilled
1 tablespoon fresh lemon juice
Angostura bitters
1 kiwi
Fresh mint leaves

Liquefy the strawberries in a food processor or blender. Halve the melon and scoop out seeds. Using a melon baller, scoop out 10–12 balls of melon flesh; cover and refrigerate.

Using a large spoon, remove the rest of the melon flesh from the rind. Peel and pit the mango. Purée the melon and mango flesh with the strawberry pulp, and strain. Flavor the soup with lemon juice and a few drops of the bitters. Ladle into two chilled bowls.

Peel and thinly slice the kiwi into medallions. Float in the soup, along with the melon balls. Garnish with mint leaves.

Pineapple Parfait Serves 4

Dates offer a sweet dose of high fiber with plenty of iron and potassium.

2 cups chopped fresh pineapple
1 cup frozen raspberries, thawed
1 cup vanilla soy yogurt
1 firm, medium banana, peeled and sliced
⅓ cup chopped dates
¼ cup sliced almonds, toasted

In sundae glasses, layer pineapple, raspberries, yogurt, banana, and dates. Sprinkle almonds over the top.

Dynamic Duo: Date & Pineapple Serves 2

You've got a date with a pineapple—literally. The combo supplies pineapple's digestive enzymes and energy-boosting manganese with dates' high fiber, potassium, and iron. The kiwi adds fiber and packs in vitamin C as well.

½ small fresh pineapple
1 kiwi
4 fresh dates
1 tablespoon fresh lime juice, including pulp
1 tablespoon plus 2 teaspoons floral honey
1 tablespoon toasted coconut
2 teaspoons ground flaxseeds

Cut off the pineapple rind from the sides, removing as much of the "eyes" as possible. Slice fruit lengthwise into quarters and remove the core. Cut into slices, reserving the juice. Peel and slice the kiwi into medallions. Remove the dates' pits and chop dates into segments. Stir together the lime and pineapple juices and honey. Toss juice and fruit mixtures and sprinkle with coconut and flaxseeds.

Dynamic Duo II: Kiwi & Strawberry Serves 2

It's no secret that kiwis and strawberries make a fine team, too. And the pair's fiber and vitamin C content is off the charts.

½ lime
1 tablespoon maple syrup
Dash of vanilla
8 ounces small, fresh strawberries
2 kiwis
1–2 tablespoons chopped pecans

Thoroughly rinse and dry the lime, grate its zest, and squeeze its juice. Stir zest and juice with maple syrup and vanilla. Gently rinse and hull the strawberries, and cut into thick slices. Peel and slice the kiwi into medallions.

Arrange the fruit on dessert plates, drizzle with syrup, and sprinkle with pecans.

Fruited Quinoa Serves 6

Whole grains such as quinoa are good sources of phytoestrogens, plant compounds that may affect blood cholesterol levels, blood vessel elasticity, bone metabolism, and many other cellular metabolic processes.

¾ cup hot water
⅛ teaspoon salt
½ cup quinoa
¼ cup mango juice concentrate, thawed
1 tablespoon white wine vinegar
1 ½ teaspoons xylitol
½ teaspoon grated orange peel
½ cup blueberries
½ cup hulled, halved strawberries
½ cup peach chunks
½ cup plum chunks
Fresh mint leaves for garnish

In a 1 quart saucepan, bring water to a boil with the pinch of salt. Add quinoa, stir, and cook on low for 10–15 minutes, until all liquid is absorbed. Transfer quinoa to a medium-sized mixing bowl, fluff lightly with fork, and set aside.

In a small bowl, combine mango juice concentrate, vinegar, xylitol, and orange zest. Blend well with a wire whisk. Add half the mango mixture to the quinoa and mix well. Cover and chill at least 1 hour.

Add remaining mango mixture and remaining ingredients to quinoa. Toss gently to combine. Garnish with mint leaves.

Your-Favorite-Fruit Dessert

Nothing scores higher on the detox scale than fiber-rich, base-forming foods, such as fresh fruit, for dessert. Eat it raw as often as possible, because cooking destroys some nutrients. I recommend fresh pineapple, rich in protein-digesting bromelain and energy-producing manganese. Or enjoy a wedge of melon, a bowl of berries, slivers of a shiny apple, a sliced banana drizzled with honey, a small bunch of juicy grapes, a handful of cherries—or perhaps you're ready for a naked papaya!

pH of Common Foods

The values listed here are for the foods in their natural state. Some have slightly different effects on your body after they are digested, but this will give you an idea. The foods are listed by:

Acidic (pH from 1.0–4.6)	Moderately Acidic (pH from 3.1–5.5)	Less Acidic and More Alkaline (pH from 5.5–10.0)
Beverages		
Ginger ale (2.0–4.0)	Beer (4.0–5.0)	Mineral water (6.2–9.4)
Lime juice (2.2–2.4)	Coffee (4.9–5.2)	Distilled water (6.8–7.0)
Lemon juice (2.2–2.6)		
Wine (2.3–3.8)		
Cranberry juice (2.5–2.7)		
Cider (2.9–3.3)		
Grapefruit juice (2.9–3.4)		
Currant juice (3.0)		
Orange juice (3.0–4.0)		
Apple juice (3.3–3.5)		
Pineapple juice (3.4–3.7)		
Prune juice (3.7–4.3)		
Tomato juice (3.9–4.3)		
Fruit		
Lime (1.8–2.0)	Peach (3.1–4.7)	Papaya (5.2–5.7)
Lemon (2.2–2.4)	Cherries (3.2–4.7)	Persimmon (5.4–5.8)
Cranberry sauce (2.3)	Pear (3.4–4.7)	Avocado (5.5–6.0)
Orange (2.8–4.2)	Mango (3.9–4.6)	Dates (6.2–6.4)
Plum (2.8–4.6)	Asian pear (4.2–4.6)	Cantaloupe (6.2–6.5)
Rhubarb (2.9–3.4)	Banana (4.5–5.2)	Melon (6.3–6.7)
Apple (2.9–3.5)	Figs (4.6–5.0)	
Raspberries (2.9–3.7)		
Grapefruit (2.9–4.0)		
Boysenberries (3.0–3.3)		
Grapefruit (3.0–3.5)		
Strawberries (3.0–4.2)		
Blackberries (3.0–4.2)		
Blueberries (3.2–3.6)		
Pineapple (3.2–4.1)		
Kiwi (3.3–3.8)		
Applesauce (3.4–3.5)		
Apricots (3.5–4.0)		
Raisins (3.6–4.2)		

Acidic (pH from 1.0–4.6)	Moderately Acidic (pH from 3.1–5.5)	Less Acidic and More Alkaline (pH from 5.5–10.0)
Vegetables & Beans		
Sauerkraut (3.1–3.7)	Tomato (3.7–4.9)	Sweet pepper (4.8–6.0)
Cucumber (3.1–3.8)	Eggplant (4.5–4.7)	Spinach (4.8–6.8)
	String beans (4.6)	Carrot (4.9–6.3)
	Pumpkin (4.8–5.5)	Asparagus (5.0–6.1)
	Squash (5.0–5.4)	Turnip (5.2–5.6)
		Cabbage (5.2–6.3)
		Broccoli (5.2–6.5)
		Sweet Potato (5.3–5.6)
		Onion (5.3–5.8)
		Peas (5.3–6.8)
		Turnip greens (5.4–5.6)
		White potato (5.4–6.3)
		Artichoke (5.6)
		Cauliflower (5.6–6.7)
		Parsley (5.7–6.0)
		Celery (5.7–6.1)
		Corn (5.9–7.3)
		Lettuce (6.0–6.4)
		Mushrooms (6.0–6.5)
		Brussels sprouts (6.3–6.6)
		Baked beans (4.8–5.5)
		Dried beans (4.9–5.5)
		Kidney beans (5.2–5.4)
		Lima beans (5.4–6.5)
		Soybeans (6.0–6.6)
Nuts & Seeds		
		Walnuts (5.4–5.5)
		Almonds (>6.0)
		Flaxseeds (>6.0)
		Hazelnuts (>6.0)
		Pecans (>6.0)
		Poppy seeds (>6.0)
		Pumpkin seeds (>6.0)
		Sesame seeds (>6.0)
		Sunflower seeds (>6.0)

Acidic (pH from 1.0–4.6)	Moderately Acidic (pH from 3.1–5.5)	Less Acidic and More Alkaline (pH from 5.5–10.0)
Red Meat		
	Dry Sausage (4.4–5.6)	Beef (5.3–6.2) Pork (5.3–6.4) Hot dogs (6.2)
Fish & Shellfish		
		Halibut (5.5–5.8) Sardines (5.7–6.6) Tuna (5.9–6.1) Mackerel (5.9–6.2) Oysters (5.9–6.7) Clams (5.9–7.1) Salmon (6.1–6.5) Haddock (6.2–6.7) Catfish (6.6–7.0) Scallops (6.8–7.1) Crab (6.8–8.0) Shrimp (6.8–8.2)
Poultry		
		Chicken and turkey (5.5–6.4) Duck (6.0–6.1) Egg yolk (6.0–6.3) Egg white (7.9–9.5)
Condiments & Seasonings		
	Fermented vegetables (3.9–5.1) Red pimento (4.3–5.2)	Hot peppers (4.8–6.0) Garlic (5.3–6.3) Cocoa (5.5–6.0) Ripe, canned olives (5.9–7.3) Dutch processed chocolate (7.0–8.0)

Acidic (pH from 1.0–4.6)	Moderately Acidic (pH from 3.1–5.5)	Less Acidic and More Alkaline (pH from 5.5–10.0)
Dairy Products		
Yogurt (3.8–4.2)	Cottage cheese (4.1–5.4)	Most cheeses (5.0–6.1)
	Roquefort cheese (4.7–4.8)	Parmesan cheese (5.2–5.3)
		Evaporated milk (5.9–6.3)
		Whole cow's milk (6.0–6.8)
		Butter (6.1–6.4)
Grains		
		Wheat (>6.0)
		Rice (>6.0)
		Barley (>6.0)
		Oats (>6.0)
		Rye (>6.0)
		Millet (>6.0)
		Quinoa (>6.0)
		Amaranth (>6.0)
		Hominy (6.9–7.9)
Sweeteners		
Fruit jellies (3.0–3.5)		Molasses (5.0–5.4)
Fruit jams (3.5–4.0)		Honey (6.0–6.8)
		Maple syrup (6.5–7.0)

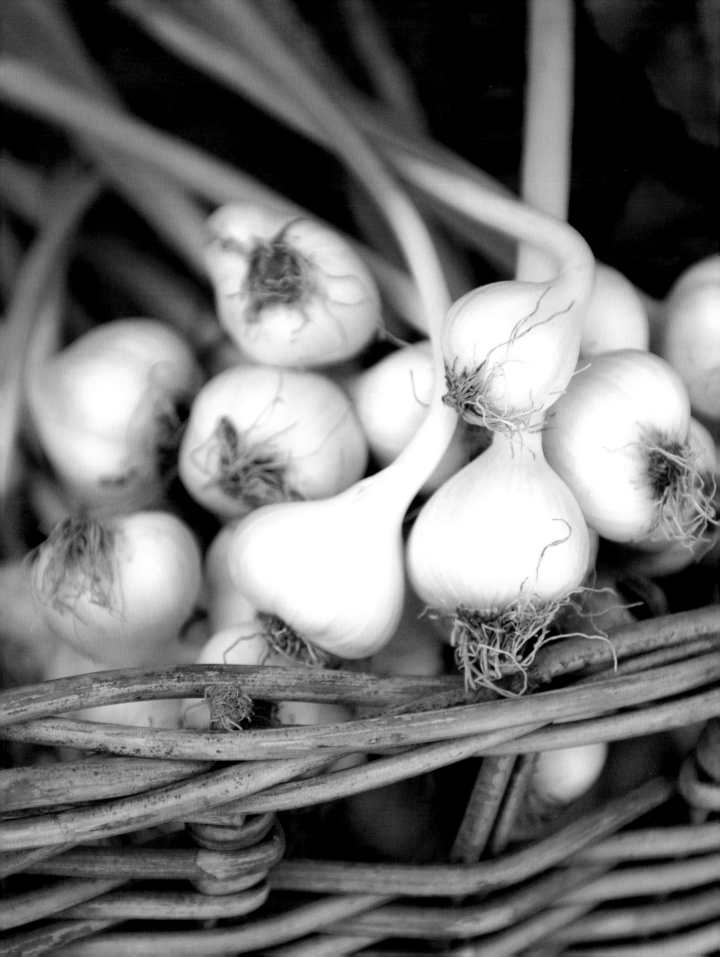

Index

A

Acidic body, 13–15
Alcohol, 17–18, 25, 82, 189
Alkaline body, 16–17
Almonds, 90, 99, 141
   Muesli with Diced Mango and Figs, 43
Aloe vera, 25
   Mango-Aloe Soother, 33
Alpha-carotene, 141, 156
Alpha linolenic acid, 110
Amaranth-Vegetable Stir-Fry, 62
American College for the Advancement of
   Medicine, 83
Anti-inflammatory foods, 83–84, 105, 108,
   113, 140, 182, 189
Antioxidants, 25, 27, 44, 47, 71, 72, 76, 84,
   140, 141, 181, 191
Aphrodisiac, natural, 140, 154
Appetizers. *See Snacks & Appetizers*
Apple(s), 140, 152
   Buckwheat-, Granola, 45
   Cabbage and, Slaw, 174
   -Cinnamon Quinoa "Cake," 134
   Mango, & Ginger Smoothie, 154
   pectin, 121, 140
   Smoked Salmon on Mock Rye with,
   -Horseradish Spread, 108
   Svelte Waldorf Salad, 121
   -of-Your-Eye Pancakes, 44
Apricot(s), 31
   Corn Flake Muffins, 35
   -Nut Smoothie, 31
   Stewed, 171
Aromatherapy, 89
Artichokes, 152
   Cherry Tomato Salad with, Hearts, 115
   with Sorrel & Radish Dips, 158
   Steamed, with Avocado Dip, 38
   Tangy, Dip, 163

Arugula
   Asparagus & Greens Salad, 172
   Pâté, 99
Asparagus
   & Greens Salad, 172
   and Herb Omelet, 166
   Lux Lox Soup, 178
   Turkey with Marinated, 123
   Turkey-Wrapped & Basil-Dipped, 105
Aspartic acid, 166
Avocado, 32
   Chicken Stir-Fry with, 63
   Fruit Shake, 32
   Steamed Artichokes with, Dip, 38

B

Baking soda, 111
Banana
   Black Currant-, Blend, 32
   BoysenNana Smoothie, 154
   -Hazelnut Muffins, 36
   Hot Cereal and Flax with, Topping, 50
   "Ice Cream," 71
Basil, Turkey-Wrapped &, -Dipped
   Asparagus, 105
Bean(s), 152
   Dip with Leeks, 37
   Fettuccine Alfredo, 125
   Lemon Shrimp with Three, Salad, 184
   Tex-Mex Red, Salad, 122
Beauty quick tips, 55
Bee pollen
   Mocha Shake, 34
Berries, 143, 152
   Mixed, Pistachio Parfait, 107
   Risotto with Melon Purée and, 49
   Sunshine Muesli, 51
   Very Berry Jam, 114

   with Yogurt Cream, 191
   See also specific berries
Beta-carotene, 26, 33, 34, 107, 140, 143
Bicarbonate boost, 15, 17
Bioflavonoids, 169, 191
Blackberry
   Fool, 168
   Sorbet, 136
   Sorbet Float, 71
Blueberries
   Waffles with, 51
Bone health, 17, 43, 50, 55, 143, 191
Boysenberries
   BoysenNana Smoothie, 154
Bread
   Potato-Spelt, 111
   Whole-Grain, with Very Berry Jam, 114
Breakfast
   Almond Muesli with Diced Mango and
   Figs, 43
   Apple-of-Your-Eye Pancakes, 44
   Asparagus and Herb Omelet, 166
   Baked Oatmeal, 165
   Blackberry Fool, 168
   bountiful cold options, 52
   Broccoli Frittata, 106
   Brown Rice & Celery Root Griddle-
   cakes with Herbed Yogurt, 169
   Buckwheat-Apple Granola, 45
   Cereal Flakes with Peaches, 46
   Fruit Eye Opener, 170
   Fruit Salad with Buckwheat and
   Seeds, 47
   Hot Cereal and Flax with Banana
   Topping, 50
   Mixed Berry Pistachio Parfait, 107
   No-Cook Red Currant-Strawberry
   Jam, 107
   Oat Porridge, 170
   Poached Huevos Rancheros, 110

Potato-Spelt Bread, 111
Risotto with Melon Puree and
    Berries, 49
Smoked Salmon on Mock Rye with
    Apple-Horseradish Spread, 108
Stewed Apricots, 171
Sunshine Muesli, 51
Tortilla Española, 113
Waffles with Blueberries, 51
Warm Wake-Up Cereal, 171
Whole-Grain Bread with Very
    Berry Jam, 114
Breast cancer protection, 42, 53, 99, 141, 187
Broccoli, 141, 152
    Frittata, 106
    -Sauerkraut Salad, 53
Bromelain, 59, 84, 83. *See also Pineapple*
Buckwheat
    -Apple Granola, 45
    Fruit Salad with, and Seeds, 47
Burritos, Tofu, 188

C

Cabbage, 152
    and Apple Slaw, 174
    See also Sauerkraut
Caffeine, 14, 18–19, 25, 168
    coffee substitutes, 14, 19
Calcium, 55, 68, 71, 107, 136, 141, 143,
    152, 158, 170, 184
Cancer-fighting foods, 5, 53, 99, 113, 140,
    141, 142, 143, 156, 165, 182, 187
Candida fungus (yeast infection), 18, 20
Carotenoids, 49, 54, 127, 141, 142
Carrot, 141, 152
    & Mango Blend, 156
    Mango-, Cocktail, 33
    Red Lentils with, -Spinach Confetti, 57
Cashew, Pineapple Stew, 186
Celery, 152
Celery root (celeriac), 98, 169
    Brown Rice &, Griddlecakes with Her-
    bed Yogurt, 169

Spicy Veggie Cocktail, 98
Cereal
    Almond Muesli with Diced Mango and
        Figs, 43
    Baked Oatmeal, 165
    Buckwheat-Apple Granola, 45
    Flakes with Peaches, 46
    Hot, and Flax with Banana Topping, 50
    Oat Porridge, 170
    Sunshine Muesli, 51
    Warm Wake-Up, 171
Cervical dysplasia, 140
Chicken
    Asian, and Brown Rice, 124
    Chinese, Soup, 175
    Kabobs with Radi-Cumber Salad, 116
    and Papaya Kebabs, 181
    Stir-Fry with Avocado, 63
Chiles, 152
Chives, Mashed Potatoes with Herring,
    Radishes, &, 183
Chocolate, 140
    Mocha Shake, 34
    Pudding, 72
    Strawberries with, & Vanilla Dips, 139
    substitute, 20
Choline, 54
Chromium, 86, 90, 124
Coconut, 189
    Turkey in, Milk with Wild Rice, 189
Condiments, 14, 16, 18
Cookies
    Pumpkin, 75
    Pumpkin Oatmeal, 138
Copper, 26, 107, 111, 141, 143, 170,
    179, 186
Cornmeal Johnnycakes with Radish
    Salad, 162
Cucumber
    Chicken Kabobs with Radi-Cumber
        Salad, 116
    Chilly Dilly, Concoction, 92
Cumin-Get-It Popcorn, 102
Currants
    Black, -Banana Blend, 32
    No-Cook Red, -Strawberry Jam, 107
Cyranine, 38

D

Dates
    Chocolate Pudding, 72
    Dynamic Duo: Pineapple &, 194
Dehydrating foods, 25
Dental cavities, preventing, 75
Dessert
    Apple-Cinnamon Quinoa "Cake," 134
    Banana "Ice Cream," 71
    Baked Pears, 136
    Basque Fruit Compote, 190
    Berries with Yogurt Cream, 191
    Blackberry Sorbet, 136
    Blackberry Sorbet Float, 71
    Chilled Fruit Soup, 135
    Chocolate Pudding, 72
    Dynamic Duo: Date & Pineapple, 194
    Dynamic Duo II: Kiwi &
        Strawberry, 194
    Fresh Fruit Kabobs, 73
    Fruited Quinoa, 195
    Maplenut Sundae, 73
    MeloMango & KiwiBerry Soup, 193
    Papaya Soup, 139
    Pineapple Parfait, 193
    Plum Dumplings, 76
    Pumpkin Cookies, 75
    Pumpkin Oatmeal Cookies, 138
    Strawberries with Chocolate & Vanilla
        Dips, 139
    Yum Yam Frosting, 77
Detoxification, 6, 9, 145–52
    dry brush massage, 151
    emotional, 150–51
    foods for, 37, 49, 73, 152
    love-your-liver program, 148–51
    nutrients for, 38
Diary products, 18, 19, 40
Diindolylmenthane (DIM), 141
Diuretic, natural, 99, 166, 169
Dinner
    Amaranth-Vegetable Stir-Fry, 62
    Asian Chicken and Brown Rice, 124
    Boiled Potatoes with Creamy Sauce, 64
    Chicken and Papaya Kebabs, 181

Chicken Stir-Fry with Avocado, 63
Fettuccine Alfredo, 125
Fish in Dill Sour Cream, 182
Fish Stew, 65
Garbanzo Shepherd's Pie, 126
Hawaiian Grilled Salmon Salad with
    Tropical Fruit Salsa, 127
Lemon Shrimp with Three-Bean
    Salad, 184
Mashed Potatoes with Herring,
    Radishes, & Chives, 183
New England-Style Chowder, 66
Niçoise Salad, 67
Pineapple Cashew Stew, 186
Portobello Quiche, 187
Quinoa-Stuffed Zucchini, 129
Sautéed Shrimp & Vegetables, 130
Stir-Fried Garbanzos & Green
    Vegetables, 132
Stir-Fried Halibut with Vegetables, 68
Thai Tilapia, 133
Tofu Burritos, 188
Turkey in Coconut Milk with Wild
    Rice, 189
Turkey and Endive Salad, 70
Dips
    Avocado, 38
    Bean, with Leeks, 37
    Sorrel & Radish, 158
    Tangy Artichoke, 163
    Turkey and Herb, with Crudités, 104

E

Eating out, 21
Edamame, 140
EFAs (essential fatty acids), 26, 27, 41, 32,
    36, 40, 41, 83, 115, 141, 142, 183
    hair and, 26, 28
    health benefits, 27
    Omega-3 or Omega-6 fats, 40, 50, 58,
    66, 73, 83, 110
    skin and, 27
Egg(s)
    Asparagus and Herb Omelet, 166

Broccoli Frittata, 106
    Chopped, and Tuna Sandwich, 54
    Poached Huevos Rancheros, 110
Endive
    Turkey and, Salad, 70
Energy, 6, 66, 93, 173, 175, 191, 194
Enzymes
    detoxifying, 140
    digestive, 82, 83, 95, 96, 103, 139, 194
    supplement for, 84
Eye health, 6, 55, 127, 141, 142

F

Fasting, 150
Fats, saturated, 127
Fennel, 152
Fettuccine Alfredo, 125
Fiber, 41, 50, 66, 71, 92, 101, 102, 113,
    122, 125, 126, 136, 138, 141, 143, 152,
    170, 181, 184, 193, 194
Fig(s)
    Almond Muesli with Diced Mangos
    and, 43
Fish, 14, 16, 152
    in Dill Sour Cream, 182
    New England-Style Chowder, 66
    Stew, 65
    Stir-Fried Halibut with Vegetables, 68
    Thai Tilapia, 133
Flavonoids, 47
Flax
    BoysenNana Smoothie, 154
    Hot Cereal and, with Banana
    Topping, 50
    Pear & Kiwi Smoothie, 155
Flaxseed, 140
    oil, 83, 110
Folic acid, 33, 71, 93, 123, 140, 181, 184
Food allergies, 19, 20, 82, 142
Food diary, 83
Food substitutions, 83
Frosting, Yum Yam, 77
Fruit, 14, 16, 152, 173
    Basque, Compote, 190

Chilled, Soup, 135
    as dessert, 195
    Eye Opener, 170
    Fresh, Kabobs, 73
    Quinoa, 195
    Salad with Buckwheat and Seeds, 47
    Tropical, Salsa, 103
    See also specific fruits

G

Gamma-linoleic acid, 45
Garbanzo beans (chickpeas), 90, 141
    Hummus, 101
    Shepherd's Pie, 126
    Stir-Fried, & Green Vegetables, 132
Gazpacho, 118
Ginger, 141, 152
    Apple, Mango, &, Smoothie, 154
    Chinese Chicken Soup, 175
    -Tumeric Toddy, 156
Glutathione peroxidase, 140
Glutathione S-transferase, 140
GORP Deluxe, 163
Grains, 14, 16, 114, 138, 152, 170, 173
    amaranth, 62
    quinoa, 129, 134, 142, 179, 195
    spelt, 111
    unrefined, 143
Granola, Buckwheat-Apple, 45
Grapefruit
    Red Lentils with Carrot-Spinach
    Confetti, 57
Grapes, 152
    Fruit Salad with Buckwheat and Seeds, 47
Green tea, 47, 84, 90, 156
    iced, 140
    Iced Peachy, 95

H

Hazelnut, Banana-, Muffins, 36
Herring, Mashed Potatoes with, Radishes,
    & Chives, 183

Honey, 20, 139
    Mango Lassi, 93
    Mocha Shake, 34
    No-Cook Red Currant-Strawberry
        Jam, 107
    Papaya Soup, 139
Hair, 6, 7, 8–9, 26, 28, 55, 67
Heart health, 5, 17, 18, 32, 41, 47, 55, 66,
    71, 106, 113, 119, 125, 143, 165, 183
Herb
    Asparagus and, Omelet, 166
    Brown Rice & Celery Root Griddle-
        cakes with, Yogurt, 169
    Turkey and, Dip with Crudités, 104
Horseradish, Smoked Salmon on Mock
    Rye with Apple-, Spread, 108
Hummus, 101, 140

I

Immune boosters, 77, 143, 165, 189
Internet sources
    author's website, 21, 83
    healthyshopping.com, 72
    pH Choice, 21
    physician locator, 83
Inulin, 172
Iodine, 68
Iron, 40, 68, 72, 76, 99, 107, 141, 143, 184,
    193, 194
Isoflavones, 140, 155

J

Jam
    No-Cook Red Currant-Strawberry, 107
    Very Berry, 114
Johnnycakes, Cornmeal, with Radish
    Salad, 162

K

Kava, 141
    Sweet Dreams Tea, 97

Kiwi
    Dynamic Duo II: Strawberry &, 194
    MeloMango & KiwiBerry Soup, 193
    Pear &, Smoothie, 155
    Strawberry &, Minty Milkshake, 97

L

L-carnitine, 84–85
L-phenylamine, 90, 132
L-tyrosine, 85, 90, 104, 116, 139
Legumes, 14, 16, 173
Lentils
    East Indian, Soup, 177
    Red, with Carrot-Spinach Confetti, 57
Lettuce, 127, 140, See also Salad
Lignans, 143
Liver health, 9, 82, 145–52, 189
Lutein, 127, 141, 143
Lycopene, 60, 140, 142

M

Magnesium, 43, 46, 60, 71, 92, 107, 136,
    141, 143, 154, 158, 159, 170, 171, 173,
    179, 181, 183, 184
Manganese, 111, 138, 143, 170, 194
Mango, 140
    Almond Muesli with Diced, and Figs, 43
    -Aloe Soother, 33
    Apple, & Ginger Smoothie, 154
    Carrot &, Blend, 156
    -Carrot Cocktail, 33
    Lassi, 93
    MeloMango & KiwiBerry Soup, 193
    Persimmon-, Cooler, 34
    Tropical Tofu Smoothie, 155
Mannoheptulose, 32
Maple syrup
    Maplenut Sundae, 73
Margarine substitute, 18
Meat, 14, 16, 18, 85, 152
Melon, 141

Chilled Fruit Soup, 135
    MeloMango & KiwiBerry Soup, 193
    Risotto with, Purée and Berries, 49
Menopause and menopausal
    symptoms, 17, 18, 24
Menstrual problems and PMS, 5, 17, 18,
    19, 77, 120, 143
Mental clarity, 6, 12, 54, 66, 93, 132, 140
Metabolic type (acidic or alkaline), 13–15
Metabolism boosters, 84–85, 90, 99, 115,
    116, 132
Miso Soup, 119
Molybdenum, 122
MSM (methylsulfonylmethane), 83
Muffins
    Apricot Corn Flake, 35
    Banana-Hazelnut, 36
    Brown Rice, 159
Mushroom(s)
    Portobello Quiche, 187
    Turkey Prosciutto-, Appetizer, 42
Mustard, 59

N

Nails (finger and toe), healthy, 44, 55
Nausea remedy, 140, 154
Nut(s), 107, 141, 152, 173
    Apricot-, Smoothie, 31
    See also specific types

O

Oatmeal, oat bread or oat flour
    Apple-of-Your-Eye Pancakes, 44
    Baked Oatmeal, 165
    Porridge, 170
    Pumpkin, Cookies, 138
    Tuna Cream on, Toast, 41
Olive oil, 106, 115, 142
Olives
    Pepita Salsa Verde, 40
Onion, 113
    Tortilla Española, 113

P

Pancakes
  Apple-of-Your-Eye, 44
  Brown Rice & Celery Root Griddle-
    cakes with Herbed Yogurt, 169
Pantothetic acid, 31, 181
Papaya, 83, 103, 142
  Chicken and, Kebabs, 181
  Naked, Breeze, 93
  Soup, 139
Paprika, 152
Pasta
  Fettuccine Alfredo, 125
  wheat substitutes for, 20
Peaches
  Cereal Flakes with, 46
  Iced Peachy Green Tea, 95
Pea(s), 152
Peanuts
  GORP Deluxe, 163
Pear(s), 152
  Baked, 136
  & Kiwi Smoothie, 155
Pecan(s)
  Svelte Waldorf Salad, 121
Pepper, 152
Peppers, bell
  Pineapple Salsa, 160
  Quesadillas with Salsa, 120
Persimmon-Mango Cooler, 34
pH balance
  ABCs of super health and glowing
    beauty, 140–43
  acidifying American diet and, 7, 13
  aging and acidic body pH, 8
  alkalinizing food choices, 8, 14
  beauty benefits, 5, 6
  bicarbonate supplement, 15, 17
  body's buffering system and, 7–8, 12,
    16–17
  bone health and, 17
  buffer burnout, 17
  chart of common foods, 196–201
  food substitutes of alkaline diet, 18
  health benefits, 5, 8–9

healthy state, pH for, 12
high alkaline producing individuals, 7, 16
hormone supplements and, 17
rejuvenation, 5
self-test, 13
symptoms of imbalance, 17
pH Choice, 21
Phenols, 76, 97
Phenylethylamine, 90, 99
Phosphorus, 55, 102, 107, 141
Phytoestrogens, 195
Pineapple, 83
  Bell Pepper, Salsa, 160
  Cashew Stew, 186
  Dynamic Duo: Date &, 194
  Naked Papaya Breeze, 95
  Parfait, 193
  Strawberry Cooler, 96
  Sunshine Muesli, 51
  Tropical Tofu Smoothie, 155
Pistachio, Mixed Berry, Parfait, 107
Plum Dumplings, 76
Polyphenols, 72, 84, 90, 95, 140
Popcorn, Cumin-Get-It, 102
Potassium, 42, 43, 50, 55, 60, 71, 71, 72,
  92, 102, 107, 136, 138, 141, 143, 152,
  154, 158, 159, 166, 170, 171, 172, 173,
  179, 181, 183, 193, 194
Potato(es), 152
  Baked, Chips, 159
  Boiled, with Creamy Sauce, 64
  Garbanzo Shepherd's Pie, 126
  Plum Dumplings, 76
  -Spelt Bread, 111
  Tortilla Española, 113
Poultry, 14, 16. See also Chicken; Turkey
Prostaglandins, 82–83, 141
Protein, 14, 33, 54, 55, 58, 62, 64, 101,
  129, 130, 141
Pterostilbene, 47
Pumpkin
  Cookies, 75
  Cream Soup, 56
  Oatmeal Cookies, 138
Pumpkin seeds (Pepita)
  Pepita Salsa Verde, 40

Q

Quercetin, 44, 83–84, 108, 113, 140
Quesadillas with Salsa, 120
Quiche, Portobello, 187
Quinoa, 134, 143
  Apple-Cinnamon, "Cake," 134
  Fruited, 195
  Salad, 179
  -Stuffed Zucchini, 129

R

Radicchio
  Fish Stew, 65
Radish(es)
  Artichokes with Sorrel &, Dips, 158
  Chicken Kabobs with Radi-Cumber
    Salad, 116
  Cornmeal Johnnycakes with, Salad, 162
  Mashed Potatoes with Herring, &
    Chives, 183
Raisins
  GORP Deluxe, 163
Raspberry, 143
  Vinaigrette, 180
Rice
  Asian Chicken and Brown, 124
  brown, 90, 124, 152
  Brown, & Celery Root Griddlecakes
    with Herbed Yogurt, 169
  Brown, Muffins, 159
  Risotto with Melon Purée and Berries, 49
  Turkey in Coconut Milk with Wild, 189
  Wild, with Raspberry Vinaigrette, 180
Royal jelly, 24

S

Salad
  Asparagus & Greens, 172
  Broccoli-Sauerkraut, 53
  Cherry Tomato, with Artichoke
    Hearts, 115
  Chicken Kabobs with Radi-Cumber, 116

Cornmeal Johnnycakes with Radish, 162
Hawaiian Grilled Salmon, with Tropical
    Fruit Salsa, 127
Lemon Shrimp with Three-Bean, 184
Niçoise, 67
Quinoa, 179
Smoked Salmon, 59
Svelte Waldorf, 121
Tex-Mex Red Bean, 122
Turkey and Endive, 70
Salmon, 142
    Hawaiian Grilled, Salad with Tropical
        Fruit Salsa, 127
    Lux Lox Soup, 178
    SeaBear brand, 142
    Smoked, on Mock Rye with Apple-
        Horseradish Spread, 108
    Smoked, Salad, 59
    Watercress Sandwich, 58
Salsa
    Bell Pepper Pineapple, 160
    Pepita, Verde, 40
    Quesadillas with, 120
    Tropical Fruit, 103
Sandwiches
    Chopped Egg and Tuna, 54
    Salmon Watercress, 58
Sauerkraut, 53
    Broccoli-, Salad, 53
Seeds, 173
    Fruit Salad with Buckwheat and, 47
    GORP Deluxe, 163
    Warm Wake-Up Cereal, 171
Selenium, 28, 42, 44, 58, 66, 116, 130, 152
Serotonin, 32, 114
Sex drive, 104, 132
Shakes and drinks
    Apple, Mango, & Ginger Smoothie, 154
    Apricot-Nut Smoothie, 31
    Avocado Fruit Shake, 32
    Black Currant-Banana Blend, 32
    BoysenNana Smoothie, 154
    Carrot & Mango Blend, 156
    Chilly Dilly Cucumber Concoction, 92
    Ginger-Tumeric Toddy, 156
    Iced Peachy Green Tea, 95

Mango-Aloe Soother, 33
Mango-Carrot Cocktail, 33
Mango Lassi, 93
Mocha Shake, 34
Naked Papaya Breeze, 93
Pear & Kiwi Smoothie, 155
Persimmon-Mango Cooler, 34
Pineapple Strawberry Cooler, 96
Spicy Veggie Cocktail, 98
Strawberry & Kiwi Minty Milkshake, 97
substitutes for high acidic, 18
Sweet Dreams Tea, 97
Tropical Tofu Smoothie, 155
See also Water
Shepherd's Pie, Garbanzo, 126
Shrimp
    Lemon, with Three-Bean Salad, 184
    Sautéed, & Vegetables, 130
Silicic acid, 31, 44, 92
Skin
    age spots, avoiding/removing, 26
    aging, 25, 26
    aloe vera drink for, 25
    antioxidants for, 25
    dehydrating foods to avoid, 25
    detoxifying and breaking out, 7
    EFAs and, 27
    liver health and, 150
    pH balance and, 6, 8–9
    rejuvenating, 24–25
    royal jelly for, 26
    smoking and, 26
    soy for, 24
    spirulina for, 26
    sun damage, 26
Snacks & Appetizers
    almonds, 99
    Apricot Corn Flake Muffins, 35
    Artichokes with Sorrel & Radish
        Dips, 158
    Arugula Pâté, 99
    Baked Potato Chips, 159
    Banana-Hazelnut Muffins, 36
    Bean Dip with Leeks, 37
    Bell Pepper Pineapple Salsa, 159
    Brown Rice Muffins, 159

Cornmeal Johnnycakes with Radish
    Salad, 162
Cumin-Get-It Popcorn, 102
GORP Deluxe, 163
Hummus, 101
Pepita Salsa Verde, 40
Savory Zucchini Sauté, 102
Steamed Artichokes with Avocado
    Dip, 38
Tangy Artichoke Dip, 163
Tropical Fruit Salsa, 103
Tuna Cream on Oatmeal Toast, 41
Turkey and Herb Dip with Crudités, 104
Turkey Prosciutto-Mushroom
    Appetizer, 42
Turkey-Wrapped & Basil-Dipped
    Asparagus, 105
Veggie Skewers, 166
Sorbet
    Blackberry, 136
    Blackberry, Float, 71
Sorrel, Artichokes with, & Radish Dips, 158
Soup
    Chilled, Soup, 135
    Chinese Chicken, 175
    East Indian Lentil, 177
    Gazpacho, 118
    Lux Lox, 178
    Marguerite, 179
    MeloMango & KiwiBerry, 193
    Miso, 119
    Papaya, 139
    Pumpkin Cream, 56
Soy foods, 24, 90, 119
    edamame, 140
    Miso Soup, 119
    Papaya Soup, 139
    See also Tofu
Spelt, Potato-, Bread, 111
Spinach, 152
    Asparagus & Greens Salad, 172
    Red Lentils with Carrot-, Confetti, 57
Squalene, 27
Stevia, 20
Stew
    Fish, 65

Pineapple Cashew, 186
Strawberry(ies)
    with Chocolate & Vanilla Dips, 139
    Dynamic Duo II: Kiwi &, 194
    & Kiwi Minty Milkshake, 97
    MeloMango & KiwiBerry Soup, 193
    No-Cook Red Currant-, Jam, 107
    Pineapple, Cooler, 96
    Sunshine Muesli, 51
Stress, 66, 152
    reduction, 87–89
Sugar, 19–20, 25, 72, 134
    artificial sweeteners, 20
    substitutes recommended, 14, 18, 20
Sweet potatoes, 55

T

Thyroid hormones, 85, 90, 116
Tofu, 90
    Burritos, 188
    Miso Soup, 119
    Tropical, Smoothie, 155
    Turkey and Herb Dip with Crudités, 104
Tomato(es), 143
    Cherry, Salad with Artichoke Hearts, 115
    Gazpacho, 118
    Soup Marguerite, 179
    Stuffed, 60
Tortilla Española, 113
Tryptophan, 36
Tumeric, 156, 177
    Ginger-, Toddy, 156
Tuna
    Chopped Egg and, Sandwich, 54
    Cream on Oatmeal Toast, 41
    Niçoise Salad, 67
Turkey
    in Coconut Milk with Wild Rice, 189
    and Endive Salad, 70
    and Herb Dip with Crudités, 104
    with Marinated Asparagus, 123
    Prosciutto-Mushroom Appetizer, 42
    -Wrapped & Basil-Dipped
        Asparagus, 105

V

Valerian root, 142
    Sweet Dreams Tea, 97
Vanilla, 139
    Strawberries with Chocolate &, Dips, 139
Vegetables, 14, 16, 152, 173
    Amaranth-, Stir-Fry, 62
    Sautéed Shrimp &, 130
    Spicy Veggie Cocktail, 98
    Stir-Fried Garbanzos & Green, 132
    Stir-Fried Halibut with, 68
    Turkey and Herb Dip with Crudités, 104
    Veggie Skewers, 166
Vegetarian diet, 14, 173
Vinaigrette, Raspberry, 180
Vitamin A, 25, 26
    foods high in, 25, 26, 35, 37, 71, 75, 99,
        105, 107, 135, 136, 138, 141, 142,
        143, 156, 184
Vitamin B-complex, 28, 42, 58, 101,
    107, 107, 111, 141, 143, 158, 170,
    175, 179, 181
Vitamin B2, 111, 179
Vitamin B6, 64, 179, 184
Vitamin B12, 59, 68, 130
Vitamin C, 25, 26, 84
    foods high in, 25, 26, 33, 34, 37, 57, 64,
        71, 92, 99, 107, 120, 135, 138, 140,
        142, 155, 160, 184, 194
    supplement, 83, 84
Vitamin D, 66, 107, 130, 141, 142
Vitamin E, 25
    caution, 25
    foods high in, 25, 32, 36, 71, 107,
        141, 142

W

Waffles with Blueberries, 51
Walnuts, 141
    Maplenut Sundae, 73
Water, 18, 143, 149
Watercress, Salmon, Sandwich, 58
Watermelon, 140

Weight loss, 6, 9, 79–90
    anti-inflammatory foods and, 83–84,
        105, 108, 113, 140, 182, 189
    appetite curbing, 89
    blood sugar balance, 85–86, 140, 142
    chromium deficiency, 86, 90
    exercise, 86–87
    "false fat," 9, 81–84
    "false fat" symptoms, 84
    food allergens and, 82, 142
    metabolism boosters, 84–85, 90, 99,
        115, 116, 132
    stress connection, 87–89
    thyroid hormones and, 85, 90
Wheat and gluten-containing products,
    20, 45
    substitutes, 18, 20
    symptoms of intolerance, 20, 45

X, Y, Z

Xylitol, 18, 20, 75, 143

Yams, 142
    Yum Yam Frosting, 77
Yogurt
    Berries with, Cream, 191
    Brown Rice & Celery Root Griddle-
        cakes with Herbed, 169
    Mango Lassi, 93
    Maplenut Sundae, 73

Zeaxanthin, 127, 141, 143
Zinc, 26, 107, 141, 152, 179, 184
Zucchini, 143
    Mediterranean, 55
    Quinoa-Stuffed, 129
    Savory, Sauté, 102

Get Dr. Lark's Latest Health and Beauty Breakthroughs

Dear "Naked Friends,"

Dr. Lark's FREE *Women's Health Updates* are the perfect complement to *Eat Papayas Naked* and a great way to stay in touch with Dr. Lark. Delivered right to your e-mail inbox every other week, these letters from Dr. Lark are focused entirely on your beauty, health, and wellness. Not only will you get the latest health breakthroughs, you'll also receive quick and easy tips to help you stay beautiful, healthy, and vibrant.

You're Just One Click Away From…

→ Free e-mail messages with Dr. Lark's latest health news and advice.

→ Solutions for your top health concerns—including weight loss, menopause, bone health, and increased energy—that you can get started on right away.

→ Answers to difficult questions such as how to fend off sugar cravings, improve digestion, and how to choose the right multinutrient for you.

To Sign Up for your FREE *Women's Health Updates*

1. Go to *www.drlark.com/updates*
2. Enter your name and e-mail address.
3. Receive Dr. Lark's next e-letter at your e-mail address ABSOLUTELY FREE!

Project Editor: Lisa M. Tooker; Text: Susan M. Lark, M.D.; Executive Editor: Kimberly Day; Recipe Editor: Ann Beman; Art Direction and Design: Kate Berg; Photography: Lisa Kennan Photography*; Food Stylist: Agnes Pouké Halpern*; Prop Stylist: Carol Hacker, Tableprops*; Assistant Food Stylist: Jeff Larsen*

Printed in China
ISBN 1-59637- 001-7

* Photography by Lisa Keenan Photography: cover, back cover, 2, 10, 22, 27, 30, 39, 48, 52, 61, 69, 74, 78, 94, 100, 109, 112, 117, 128, 131, 137, 144, 157, 161, 167, 173, 176, 185, 192, 200.